T0321661

Traditional Chinese Medicine, Western Science, and the Fight Against Allergic Disease

Traditional Chinese Medicine, Western Science, and the Fight Against Allergic Disease

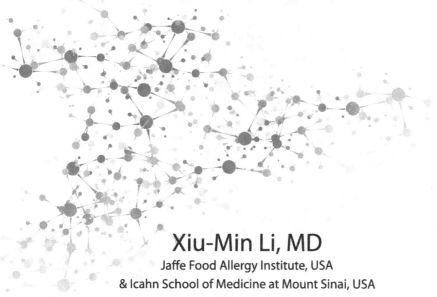

Xiu-Min Li, MD

Jaffe Food Allergy Institute, USA
& Icahn School of Medicine at Mount Sinai, USA

Henry Ehrlich

asthmaallergieschildren.com

With a special acknowledgement to:

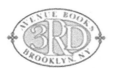

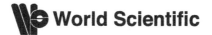 **World Scientific**

NEW JERSEY · LONDON · SINGAPORE · BEIJING · SHANGHAI · HONG KONG · TAIPEI · CHENNAI · TOKYO

Published by

World Scientific Publishing Co. Pte. Ltd.

5 Toh Tuck Link, Singapore 596224

USA office: 27 Warren Street, Suite 401-402, Hackensack, NJ 07601

UK office: 57 Shelton Street, Covent Garden, London WC2H 9HE

Library of Congress Cataloging-in-Publication Data
Names: Li, Xiumin, author. | Ehrlich, Henry, 1949–   , author.
Title: Traditional Chinese medicine, western science, and the fight against allergic disease /
    by Xiu-Min Li and Henry Ehrlich.
Description: New Jersey : World Scientific, 2016. | Includes bibliographical references and index.
Identifiers: LCCN 2015046837| ISBN 9789814733687 (hardcover : alk. paper) |
    ISBN 9789814733694 (pbk. : alk. paper)
Subjects: | MESH: Hypersensitivity--therapy | Autoimmune Diseases--therapy |
    Medicine, Chinese Traditional
Classification: LCC RC584 | NLM WD 300 | DDC 616.97--dc23
LC record available at http://lccn.loc.gov/2015046837

British Library Cataloguing-in-Publication Data
A catalogue record for this book is available from the British Library.

Copyright © 2016 by World Scientific Publishing Co. Pte. Ltd.

All rights reserved. This book, or parts thereof, may not be reproduced in any form or by any means, electronic or mechanical, including photocopying, recording or any information storage and retrieval system now known or to be invented, without written permission from the publisher.

For photocopying of material in this volume, please pay a copying fee through the Copyright Clearance Center, Inc., 222 Rosewood Drive, Danvers, MA 01923, USA. In this case permission to photocopy is not required from the publisher.

Printed in Singapore

CONTENTS

ABOUT THE AUTHORS

Xiu-Min Li, MD, is a Professor of Pediatrics in the Division of Pediatric Allergy and Immunology, at the Icahn School of Medicine at Mount Sinai. Dr. Li obtained her MD degree at the Henan School of Chinese Medicine (Zhengzhou) in 1983 and a Master's degree in Clinical Pediatric Immunology from the Graduate School of the China Academy of Chinese Medical Sciences (Beijing). She was a Visiting Scientist at Stanford and postdoctoral fellow in Clinical Immunology at Johns Hopkins where she was appointed Instructor in 1997. Dr. Li joined the Division of Pediatric Allergy and Immunology at Mount Sinai when it was established in 1997. She has chaired prominent committees about the use of alternative medicines for allergic diseases in the US and internationally and was recently named Director for the new Center for Integrative Medicine for Allergies and Wellness at Mount Sinai, to bring together research and treatment on a larger scale.

Henry Ehrlich is the editor of asthmaallergieschildren.com, co-author of *Asthma Allergies Children: A Parent's Guide*, and other works of nonfiction. His most recent book was *Food Allergies: Traditional Chinese Medicine, Western Science, and the Search for a Cure* — the first book about the work of

Dr. Xiu-Min Li, lauded as "A masterful job of distilling a lot of complex material into verbiage that can be understood by the non-scientist, albeit a sharp non-scientist, and accomplished in an entertaining style," by Dr. Arnold I. Levinson, Emeritus Professor of Medicine, Perelman School of Medicine at The University of Pennsylvania. It was published by Third Avenue Books.

ACKNOWLEDGMENTS

Dr. Li thanks her colleagues and co-researchers: Hugh Sampson, MD; Kamal Srivastava, PhD; Nan Yang, PhD; Changda Liu, PhD; Ying Song, MD; Julie Wang, MD; Stacie M. Jones, MD; Jacqueline A. Pongracic, MD; Sally Noone, RN; Jaime Ross, RN; Julia A. Wisniewski, MD; Miae Oh, MD; Madhan Masilamani, PhD; Scott Sicherer, MD; Sylvan Wallenstein, PhD; Brian Schofield, JD; Sharon Hamlin; Anna Nowak-Węgrzyn, MD; Amanda Cox, MD.

She would also like to thank those who have supported her research: NIH/NCCAM Grants; FARE [Food Allergy Research and Education]; Chris Burch Fund, Alternative Medicine Clinic and Research for Asthma and Obesity; Sean Parker Foundation, ASHMI compounds for asthma and high bioavailablity IgE inhibitory compounds; The Winston Wolkoff Fund for Integrative Medicine for Allergies and Wellness (many families contributed to this fund); Lisa Yu, the Drako family, and the Rizzoto family for their kind support; also contributors to the biomarker study and to Crowdrise for hosting it. For practice assistance: Song Park; Jenny Xiao; Ming Qi Natural Heath Care Center; Comprehensive Allergy and Asthma Care; Asthma and Allergy Associates of Murray Hill.

Both authors would also like to express gratitude to Denise Zaitoon for her incisive interview with Dr. Li in her blog Healing Hacker, Susan Weissman, Selena Bluntzer, and Paul Ehrlich, MD for their support and assistance at many points during the writing of this book.

NOTES ON THE TEXT

Except for those sections signed by Dr. Xiu-Min Li and Dr. Renata Engler and the appendix, all chapters were written by me and narrated where appropriate in the first person for coherence (I hope). The crux of these chapters is to introduce Dr. Li's published papers and put the work in context. These are all footnoted. For detailed citation of certain facts, please look up the original papers referenced.

One chapter consists of a lengthy account of a single patient's experience with a "new" disease that defied mainstream treatment, but which was controlled by Dr. Li by applying the tools and principles of traditional Chinese medicine to an individual case.

Henry Ehrlich

FOREWORD

Dr. Renata J.M. Engler

On the journey through life, one's being is touched by many people and blessed occasionally by the magic that resonates with and enhances one's own journey. Dr. Xiu-Min Li is such a gift for me. Her spirit, determination and commitment to healing in a world abundant with disease, pain and suffering reflect the best in the human family and inspire her patients, her colleagues and friends. We had the particular pleasure to collaborate on a chapter about Complementary and Alternative Medicine (CAM) for the textbook chapter in *Middleton's Allergy Principles and Practice* (8th Edition, 2014). I am deeply grateful for Dr. Li's encouragement of my efforts to contribute guidelines for traditional medicine practitioners to incorporate CAM modalities into a patient-care plan, respecting patient perspectives and needs while ensuring optimization of safety as well as efficacy ("Complementary and alternative medicine for the allergist-immunologist: Where do I start?" *Journal of Allergy and Clinical Immunology* 2009; 123(2):309–316, 316.e.1–316.e.3). It is with humble gratitude that I call Dr. Li both friend and colleague. So it is both an honor and a pleasure to write this foreword to a book about her life's work.

Like Dr. Xiu-Min Li, I am an immigrant to the shores of the United States of America, and like her, I was raised in a family that understood that healing and health maintenance often required the use of all resources and wisdom, crossing through traditional Western allopathic medicine into other traditions and fonts of knowledge. As a physician trained in internal medicine and pediatric and adult allergy-immunology as well as science-based approaches, I served as a military physician for 38 years (retiring in 2013) and now continue to work in clinical research relevant to gaps in cardiovascular disease risk assessment and reduction, incorporating cardio-immunology and the drivers of systemic inflammation into protocol development at Walter Reed Bethesda. As I move into the last quarter of my life, I am eager to be a part of medicine that is focusing on disease before it is overtly expressed with a catastrophic illness or death, and healing care that embraces Dr. Leroy Hood's four P's of holistic 21st century medicine: "predictive, preventive, personalized and participatory." (P4 Medicine Institute, http://www.p4mi.org/) Dr. Li's science and practice are the embodiment of these values.

My personal journey includes extensive experience not only as a physician seeking to optimize the care of patients with complex symptoms and with no simple diagnosis or well-defined treatments but also the extreme challenges of a caregiver struggling with the many instances where a visit to an allopathic medicine provider leaves the patient (along with their loved ones) with no practical or effective help. For me personally, the experiences as a life-long caregiver of aging, war-traumatized, dying parents and in-laws, a very sick husband, and dear friends facing hopelessness in their disease journey, have taught me as much as my long medical training. I remain continually inspired and in humble admiration of the courage, sheer labor intensity and driving force behind quality caregiving largely performed by an army of unpaid family members and friends. Listening to the caregiver perspectives and needs, as they represent patients often unable to advocate for themselves, is a critical factor in the future evolution of optimized health care. Dr. Li recognized this critical value input early in her work and as a result she is so appreciated by her patients and their families, a medal of achievement and honor that is not traditionally recognized adequately.

Like Dr. Li, I have struggled with the many gaps in our knowledge and the reality that so much of what we think we know or understand today will be significantly changed or even discarded within the next 5–7 years. A position of humility and openness to new ideas, new paradigms and multi-disciplinary team efforts to improve the precision and effectiveness of our care for patients is needed. As the science of health and healing rapidly evolves to recognize the medicinal value of nutritional content and the critical microbiome (the types of bacteria living in our gut), mindfulness and stress management rather than stress-reduction alone, exercise tailored to biodiversity, sleep and the complexities of psychoneuroimmunology, the need for bridge-builders that connect the silos of knowledge and understanding, enhancing all sides of the rivers of ignorance, is ever increasing.

Dr. Li has built these bridges. As she describes so well, our challenge for the future of global health is to develop platforms that can critically evaluate best practices for the integration of great medical traditions and to ensure that no patient is given the message of abandonment or hopelessness by those with a mission to heal.

Respectfully and with deep admiration,
Renata J. M. Engler, MD
FAAAAI, FACAAI, FACP
Professor, Medicine and Pediatrics
Uniformed Services University of the Health Sciences
Bethesda, MD

INTRODUCTION

Dr. Xiu-Min Li

When I was a teenager thinking about what to do with my life, I was fortunate to have relatives who were able to counsel me wisely about my future. One uncle had taught himself Chinese medicine from a textbook and his knowledge had served him well for years. He presented me with his prized volume and said, "There is gold in this book." He also said, you must study medicine because "if you are a doctor you will always be able to find a job." His final piece of advice was to study both traditional Chinese medicine (TCM) and Western medicine. It was as if he could look far into the future and envision our present moment in which many Westerners have medical conditions that their own doctors cannot cure, and a majority of Americans have either considered consulting alternative practitioners and attempting alternative treatments, or have actually done so.

My uncle's wisdom was confirmed when I was working at the China-Japan Friendship Hospital in Beijing after completing my studies. The son of a close friend was brought in with terrible stomach problems. My colleagues said he had an infection and put him on IV antibiotics and refined amino acids for days. He continued to suffer. We really thought he would die. So I contacted my TCM mentor who was in his 70s. He listened to my description of the patient. He thought about it and said. "No more antibiotics. No more amino acids. Give him ginseng and stir-fried wheat flour paste."

We did it, and within days this little boy was normal. From then on, I promised myself that though my greatest love was for research, I would always try to reserve some of my time for helping people using the tools of TCM. I kept that promise when I arrived at the Jaffe Food Allergy Institute at the Icahn School of Medicine at Mount Sinai in New York, after time as a Visiting Scientist at Stanford and as a Fellow at Johns Hopkins in Baltimore. Dr. Hugh Sampson brought me from Hopkins to New York as part of his team.

With the agreement of my employers, I opened an independent clinic to treat recalcitrant eczema using medicines from the ancient formulary of Chinese medicine. Eczema was a good place to start because severe itching is a disruptive threat to everyday quality of life, and when there is also compulsive scratching, the skin loses its capacity to protect us against the outside world. Oozing and bleeding allow microbes that normally sit harmlessly on the skin to penetrate where they do not belong and infect the tissue. The skin loses its capacity to help regulate body temperature. As we now know, damaged infant skin can also become an induction point for exposure to food allergens that sensitize children even in homes where parents swear the child has never ingested them.

At the time, the late 1990s, managing eczema relied on a strategy of keeping the skin moist, carefully avoiding exposures to dietary and environmental triggers, and large doses of steroids. Unfortunately, this combination of avoiding triggers and steroid usage is still the rule in much of allergic medicine.

Our food allergy research at Mount Sinai was sophisticated. My team set out in an attempt to "fool the immune system" by combining gene therapy and immunotherapy. The general idea was that we could prevent allergies to peanut protein in non-allergic mice if we could coax the mouse's own cells to produce peanut protein. For the "gene therapy" part, we injected non-allergic mice with a DNA vector containing the "gene" — or DNA instruction set — to build the highly allergenic peanut protein, Ara h2. If it worked, then the Ara h2 instructions would be incorporated into the mouse's own cells and these cells in turn would begin producing the Ara h2 peanut protein. We hoped that if the mouse's own cells were manufacturing and releasing the Ara h2 peanut protein, the immune system would deem it harmless, and later fail to become allergic — the immunotherapy part. After all, why would the immune system attack a substance made by the mouse's very own cells? As a comparison in our experiment, a control set of mice received a DNA vector without the Ara h2 gene — i.e., they were treated the same as the other mice except their cells would not produce peanut protein. We expected that these mice would later become allergic to peanut protein.

Three weeks following the DNA injection, we attempted to make both sets of mice allergic to peanut protein using an established protocol that is known to make naïve mice "allergic." At this point, we did not expect either set of mice to be allergic to peanut protein. To our surprise, when we were getting ready to sensitize the mice to peanut protein, we discovered that the mice receiving the Ara h2-containing DNA vector were already highly allergic (control mice were not allergic). That was the end of a "simple" solution to food allergy. The immune system was definitely not "fooled."

I still think this is a good idea, and we are going to try it again using a modified non-toxic form of the cholera toxin adjuvant that has been shown to be safe for pregnant women and infants. We are adapting to allergies for the first time, a novel form of delivery.

At about the time we did the gene therapy experiment I attended a fundraiser for the Jaffe Institute where I sat with a number of food allergy mothers who one-by-one recounted their sad stories about raising a child with food allergies. My co-author tells this story in his previous book: I told the mothers about my work with TCM in my clinic and they expressed a wish that I would be able to achieve similar results with food allergies to those I had with eczema. Their stories convinced me as a physician scientist that I needed to do what I could for patients now, not just work on ideas that may help over ten years from now. With great courage and wisdom and above all with compassion for patients, Dr. Sampson agreed to support my work on using TCM to treat food allergies.

Traditional Chinese medicine gives us a head start because it has developed over thousands of years in response to the medical challenges of the age. It is very practical. The history gives us clues about how to treat specific symptoms. During the Tang Dynasty (618–906) there were many wars so they learned to treat open wounds. During the Qing Dynasty (1644–1906) there were many fevers. This was also the period when contact with Europe picked up and later America, which was the start of integrative medicine. White Tiger Decoction was used for fever and it had the wonder drug aspirin as well as herbs. Chinese doctors learned how to use injections and IVs. Today, Western science helps us understand how the medicines work and how to make them better. The treatments I use for eczema incorporate medications developed for damage from burns suffered in battle. Intestinal parasites have been a problem in China for thousands of years. I treated them with modern medicines when I was a barefoot doctor as a teenager, but we have herbal treatments for them, one of which became the basis for my herbal food allergy treatment.

The Dynastic age of Chinese history is over. But the new global age presents medical challenges that are as much a part of our time as wounds and infectious diseases were in earlier times. I call these "good life" diseases, such as obesity, diabetes, and allergies, of course. All these conditions have long histories, but our current age has made them much more common. The epidemics of these conditions may have started in Westernized, affluent countries, but globalization brings with it pollution, dietary changes, new medical practices, and all the other things that seem to contribute to these diseases. Good life diseases, diseases of affluence, are increasing rapidly in countries where the hygiene hypothesis was not a factor until recently.

After two decades of work, we have a good story to tell. The clinic has now evolved well beyond eczema treatment. One day a week, and occasionally more often, I am exploring clinical applications for drugs derived from the classical formulas of Chinese medicine, which informs the laboratory work at Mount Sinai, and which in turn informs the work at the clinic. We conduct the science at the highest standards our regulators demand. At the same time, we treat patients with carefully made medicines that qualify for use as supplements. That dual regulatory system gives us great flexibility because we can use them in practice-based studies that permit us to treat patients and also advance our knowledge. For example, we are studying biomarkers to help us find out if the food allergy treatments can predict passing food challenges. This study began with funds from small donors via crowdsourcing.

One important note about my practice. I stay away from the language of TCM. It is not necessary to use the same language and terminology. Some mothers read the TCM books. Some do not. And if you say, "you have a spleen *Qi* deficiency," they get very scared. They say, "What's that?" They think their child has a defective spleen or kidney or liver. That is why I do not use that vocabulary. Patients and families rarely ask about the TCM terminology/mechanisms and I do not offer them.

As for the science, the TCM vocabulary has no place in the research. In the United States and other countries, there has been some progress toward integrating two great medical traditions. Acupuncture needles now have approval as medical devices for insurance purposes, but there is no real understanding of how they work and they are accepted without relation to the larger system we call TCM.

How then do we go forward? Since a number of medical centers have established or are going to establish integrative medical centers, where acupuncturists and herbalists can team up with conventional doctors to manage pain and give the body time to heal itself, we need to find common ground. One element is commonly overlooked. I contend that mainstream doctors do not have to understand TCM in order to give their patients the benefits. And the key to that is research. As TCM practitioners, we know that our herbs are beneficial. But the regulatory system under which the Western medical system functions must show a number of things;

1 — That our treatments are **safe**. First do no harm.
2 — That they **work**.
3 — And if they work, why they **work**.

At that point, doctors will begin to use them, without ever knowing whether a disease is rising from the spleen or descending from the liver.

As my own clinic has expanded, we find that there are more and more patients who need help with conditions beyond what we began with. Eczema patients also have asthma. Many of them have food allergies, of course. Some food allergy patients also have a condition called eosinohilic esophagitis. Patients with a variety of symptoms have mast cell activation syndrome, in which the mast cells degranulate in response to many triggers including food, heat, and chemicals. There are no answers for many of these in the allopathic tool bag. Allergists, dermatologists, and pulmonologists treat the organs and the symptoms they were trained in, but they often do not address the whole patient, body and mind, which is what TCM does. I hope working together we can connect them.

TCM gives us a place to start, although obviously it does not help with the environmental degradation and other modern factors that may contribute to the epidemic. More and more patients are finding their way to my door, some through word of mouth or social media and some through referrals of physicians who only wish the best for their patients, but who have exhausted the remedies they studied. While the research for these complicated co-morbidities is not as extensive as with our work on food allergies and asthma, we are learning enough about the biology and chemistry to make some educated guesses and test them in the clinic. As my friend and colleague Scott Sicherer has said, instead of testing the effect of one molecule on another molecule as is customary in Western medicine, TCM allows us to test multiple molecules on multiple other molecules. My hope is that other researchers will begin to build on what we are learning at Sinai to lead us in novel directions. My colleagues and I have stood on the shoulders of giants going back to the Yellow Emperor. We want others to stand with us.

The future of my practice will concentrate on the complex areas where there are few clinical answers at the moment. Obviously, conventional medicine offers relief from environmental allergies using immunotherapy, antihistamines, and nasal steroids. Most cases of allergic asthma can be controlled by conscientious use of inhaled corticosteroids (ICS) and bronchodilators, although as you will read there are other variants of asthma syndrome that resist steroid treatment or are so serious that systemic steroids must be used. Even anaphylactic food allergies are being treated by non-approved forms of immunotherapy or will be by methods under study today.

I do not want to "compete" with these therapies. I want to do what others are not doing. Where there are multiple conditions, I want to treat the immune system that ties them altogether. I want to treat asthma that does not respond to steroids, and where the treatment, as well as the disease, presents a threat to the patient's state of mind, growth, energy levels, and capacity to learn. I want to treat the digestion as well as the food allergies themselves. I also want to treat conditions where the symptoms are suggestive of things we know about but the triggers and etiology are obscure, such as mast cell activation syndrome. Most of my patients are children. For many of them, the timetable for research and approval will run well into their teens. As a physician, I want to help them. As a scientist, I believe these therapies have been proven safe, that they affect the body in favorable ways, and can be made more so. As a mother, I want these children to have their childhoods.

Chapter

1

FOOD ALLERGY

Some chimpanzees, when infected with intestinal parasites, eat bitter, foul-tasting plants, which they otherwise avoid and which contain biologically active compounds that kill intestinal parasites (Joseph Narby, *The Cosmic Serpent: DNA and the Origins of Knowledge*, 1998).

I like this passage for a couple of reasons. One is that it shows how basic the impulse to use vegetation as medicine is. TCM has thousands of years of recorded history, and clearly it did not begin with the beginnings of civilization, and it did not even start with humanity. The other is that it shows how fundamental the battle is between animals and parasites, nature's extortionists. Chimps knew these little things were bad for them even if they could not see them or imagine them. They knew they were sick and they tried to do something about it. Readers of my other book about Dr. Li, *Food Allergies: Traditional Chinese Medicine, Western Science, and the Search for a Cure* know that her explorations for a food allergy treatment began with something called *Wu Mei Wan*, an old remedy for these worms that feed off people, weakening them without killing them, except for children who may not have time to develop their own defenses. In a body battling parasites, IgE and eosinophils are powerful defenses, but in our more hygienic society, they pick on the wrong targets and become our enemies.

It is a case of mistaken identity. Certain peanut proteins are very similar to those found in helminths, commonly known as parasitic worms. Likewise proteins found in dust mites and cockroaches, which are potent environmental allergens, are similar to some found in shrimp and lobster — major food allergens. The great moment of revelation came when Dr. Li was studying food allergy reactions and it dawned on her that it sounded like parasites so she dipped into the TCM trove *Classic Formulas and Strategies* and came up with *Wu Mei Wan*. As readers will also recall, in trying to decide how to deliver this medicine to patients, Dr. Li's colleagues tasted it in the form of brewed tea, as it would be taken in China. They unanimously agreed that they could not stand the taste.

When I finished writing the other book, the Phase II trial of Food Allergy Herbal Formula-2 (FAHF-2), the successor to *Wu Mei Wan*, was still in a state of equipoise. That is, the work was done but the data had not been compiled or interpreted or published.

To recap, this double-blind, randomized, placebo-controlled study enrolled 68 subjects, 12–45 years of age, with allergies to peanut, tree nut, sesame, fish, and/or shellfish. Food allergies for all study participants were confirmed at the outset by a stringent double-blind, placebo controlled food challenge (DBPCFC). Forty-six received FAHF-2 and 22 placebo. After six months of therapy, subjects underwent another DBPCFC. For those who demonstrated increases in eliciting dose, a repeat challenge was performed three months after stopping therapy.[1]

The results were disappointing to hopeful food allergy parents. There was no clinical breakthrough from this study. However, the laboratory results do suggest positive immune modulation is possible with FAHF-2. Immunological studies of the subjects' PBMCs (peripheral blood mononuclear cells) drawn at baseline and incubated with FAHF-2 and food allergen produced significantly less IL-5, greater IL-10 and increased numbers of

---

[1] Julie Wang, MD, FAAAAI; Stacie M. Jones, MD; Jacqueline A. Pongracic, MD, FAAAAI; Ying Song, MD; Nan Yang, PhD; Scott H. Sicherer, MD; Melanie M. Makhija, MD, MS; Rachel Glick Robison, MD; Erin Moshier, MS; James Godbold, PhD; Hugh A. Sampson, MD; Xiu-Min Li, MD, MS, "Safety, clinical and immunologic efficacy of a Chinese herbal medicine (FAHF-2) for food allergy," *Journal of Allergy and Clinical Immunology* 2015; 135(2), Supplement: AB234.

Tregs than untreated cells — a shift away from the allergic Th2-dominant cytokines.

While the subjects' cells tested in the lab outside of their bodies showed benefit with FAHF-2 treatment, what happened with the subjects themselves? It turns out that 44% had trouble sticking with the protocol. The real numbers of non-compliant subjects may have been higher, but the count was taken according to how many pills were returned at the conclusion of the study period. Even more pills may still be sitting in medicine cabinets in subjects' homes.

As with most studies, in retrospect, there seem to have been holes in the design. This do not mean that FAHF-2 cannot work in humans. It was asking a great deal for nearly 70 individuals ranging in age from 12, where they would have at least been subject to some element of maternal supervision, through college age and into middle age to swallow 10 pills at each of three meals during the day, i.e., 30 pills per day. They had to remember to pack their noon dose to be taken at lunch. Strict medication regimens are best practiced under the watchful eye of mothers. Moreover, six months is a very short period of time to effect a wholesale renovation of the immune system. In her clinical practice, Dr. Li projects 2–4 years duration for treatment, so six months is a drop in the bucket. According to Dr. Li,

> There are still a lot of things to learn from this trial. We think the product itself needs to be improved — if we can reduce the number of pills we can increase compliance and optimize the product.
>
> We have identified a number of bio-active compounds and are able to detect the concentrations of the compounds in blood and urine. This method will be an important means of assessing adherence. We began to generate preliminary data using this technology. We need to test more work before drawing definitive conclusions. The preliminary data showed that the compliance rate is lower than 50%, but we have to figure out if it is a true compliance issue or the GI absorption or metabolism issues.
>
> Interestingly, the preliminary data showed that if the individuals showed high enough blood concentration of the bioactive compound marker, this individual showed good clinical outcomes. This supports our in vitro study data, which shows when human immune cells are directly exposed to FAHF-2 extract there are beneficial immune modulatory effects. There are gaps of knowledge between TCM human use experience, in vivo animal model study, human in vitro study, and then finally to human in vivo study trials. Our continued work will help us fill in the gaps.

In the earlier book, I described the creation of a refined form of FAHF-2, which employs butanol (B-FAHF-2) to separate the active ingredients from the inert ones. The FDA has approved use of B-FAHF-2 for further experiments without having to go back to square one with murine models and early-phase human trials.

The test tube indicators are encouraging. Dr. Li says,

> *For several years we have been looking at which herb compounds affect IgE. We have demonstrated that human memory B-cell lines that produce IgE could remain very high, even if they are not stimulated. You put them in a good nutrition medium and they will grow and produce IgE. In a 2014 study we compared effects of FAHF-2 and B-FAHF-2 on IgE production. Both significantly reduced IgE, but B-FAHF-2 requires nearly nine times less concentration.*

B-FAHF-2 More Potently Inhibited IgE
Production than FAHF-2 *in vitro*

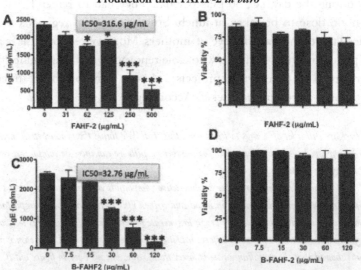

B-FAHF-2 inhibited IgE production by human memory B cells (U266 cells) at nearly 10 times lower IC50 concentration.
Yang et al. *Ann Allergy Asthma Immunol.* 2014.

> *We also screened the nine herbs from B-FAHF-2 and found three of them directly suppressed IgE. Other herbs have no direct effect on IgE, but some of them suppress inflammation and histamine release while others enhance protective immune responses such as IgG. But this study only focused on identifying the constituents*

in vitro that we focused on one of the IgE inhibitory herbs and identified the active compounds in vitro.

One of the things that make this avenue of research so exciting is that it holds out the possibility of making long-term changes in the underlying immune mechanisms. Allergic responses are "amnestic" — remembered. A patient can go years with no exposure to an allergen and then respond violently. It is this tendency that makes "avoidance" a dirty word in the food allergy community.

As Dr. Li says,

Memory cells do not need a strong stimulus, sometimes none at all. Most of the time they settle in the bone marrow where they wait until they are ready to produce IgE. We discovered the compound that regulates IgE through the modulation of one of the critical transcription factors that control IgE synthesis from memory cells.

That is the key — antibody production — that is where you use the term 'switch'. The antibody-producing B-cells can be switched in a different direction. The same cells that can produce IgG or IgE are controlled by these transcription factors. They tell this cell what to produce. And so you do not have to kill the cells; you just have to initiate the signals to control what they produce.

This is one of the few subjects that lead her to employ military metaphors. She likens it to field commanders who are getting bad orders — good soldiers implementing wrong tactics.

Lack of cytotoxicity is a crucial element. In addition, there is no suppression of innate immunity, as there is with steroids, which have the side effect of leaving patients more vulnerable to bacterial or viral infection.

This is unique finding for a natural product. They are not killing the cells. The cells can still be there, but just not produce the IgE. Also, sometimes with immunomodulation, the IgE levels are still there, only they are dormant. Then when the body needs them, they can reactivate, when you encounter an intestinal parasite, for example.

The parasite connection is fundamental.

Normally the immune system can distinguish between the different proteins — food protein is very different from bacteria. Bacteria pathogens are very different from other microbes. The cells can tell. So therefore when you get a bacterial infection, your B-cells automatically start to produce IgG. Most of the time probiotics stimulate your immune system to produce IgG. Once your immune system encounters this type of stimulus, it has the capability to produce IgG to protect the individual. But with allergies, the allergen stimulates production of IgE by B cells.

Dr. Li listens to her patients, no matter how young.

Some kids have asked me "why do we need allergy?" We are not absolutely certain yet. But you can summarize it as several things — perhaps it is a single factor or combination but it has to do with microbials. There is a short window when the fetus is in the mom's uterus when the immune system is skewed toward Th2 — but then after birth they need to gain quickly and switch to Th1 dominance through exposure to the microbials. So a type of microbial exposure is a major factor. Another theory holds that the mother or the post-natal infant is exposed to food too early or too late. This was the prevailing theory for 10–15 years, but has been recently rejected. We avoided the peanut early and the prevalence of peanut allergy (PA) has doubled. So the problem was not direct peanut exposure. Now there is no peanut restriction on mothers but the peanut prevalence allergy has tripled. We still have no consensus.

A new study is planned for B-FAHF-2 to be administered over 26 months using six pills per day instead of the 30 pills over six months. This one will be evenly divided, 17 each of medicine and placebo. While smaller, the study should produce robust data with easier compliance. This is just one of several studies using the refined food allergy formula planned over the next several years in support of the eventual aim of having a medicine that can be prescribed without accompanying knowledge of TCM. B-FAHF-2 is an FDA-registered investigational new drug (IND).

Many mothers ask if the goal of Dr. Li's food allergy treatment is to "bite proof" patients, i.e., give them protection against small inadvertent ingestion of their allergens, desensitize them to their allergens, or to cure their allergies. The goal has always been to "reeducate" the immune system to fight the things that need fighting and ignore the ones that do not with enough capacity to fight natural enemies like parasites — a cure.

Since I started working on food allergy research, we have tested many novel therapies that we thought would be effective but when we started herbal treatment the first time we saw the mice were protected. They were all protected. It was beautiful.

Of course those mice were all fed through a tube.

> *If you reach the dose and duration of the mice (100%) with people, we have a good chance. But persuading our participants to use a full dose and for a long time is a big job. This product we hope will make their efforts easier. In the new blinded trial and my practice-based biomarker study we are going to use the refined product, which I hope will point the way for the pursuit of the IND.*

What will the biochemistry show?

> *Then you'll get protection even though your IgE may not be at a normal level. That is my prediction. Reactions don't only involve IgE, but additional types of cells such as mast cells and basophils. The protection is not only due to reduction of IgE, but also induction of other antibodies such as IgA and IgG.*
>
> *When we did the animal study, before treatment, the mice had a similar IgE level as post treatment. But in the middle, before treatment commenced, we gave a boosting dose to drive their IgE levels very high. Then after treatment the IgE got lower, but never low like the level was normal or to the level before we boosted them.*
>
> *In mice, we don't do "greater than 100" which is how it's reported by laboratories for patients. For mice, we do a real level — for example 4,000 or 5,000, high enough to ensure that when we challenge them they have a reaction. And then after we boost them, their IgE level could reach 5,000. Then after treatment the 5,000 level can drop 2,000 or 2,500 or a little bit more than that, but at that time when you challenge... they don't have any reactions. Even with people we know that it's not the level of serum IgE that causes a reaction, it's the number of antibodies that are attached to effector cells via high affinity receptors.*
>
> *With very high IgE levels, if you are able to drop it to a certain level, I think you do not need it to be normal. After treatment, you may build up a new level of tolerance. In Chinese medicine, they talk about balance so I think in terms of the treatment just bringing a new level of balance. You cannot go back to baseline, like a new baby before they've been exposed to the allergens. But you can effect a switch that starts to build up a good protective immune response and bring a new balance... so they are still healthy, they don't have reactions, but not zero IgE.*

Laboratory experiments are encouraging on this score.

Recognizing the importance of IgE levels to patients and their anxious parents, Dr. Li is also working on a new herbal treatment to explicitly reduce

IgE production — one mother referred to it as "IgE tea" and the name stuck (see below).

> *You can still have IgE, but you also have lots of IgG, IgA, and many other protective antibodies. That is very good. These antibodies circulate. And for example, if you have peanut protein that gets in, they grab the protein and don't give it a chance to bind to IgE on the effector cells. These other antibodies are also specific so they can do that. So the individual will not have a reaction. The protection happens in many ways, not just dropping the IgE.*

Small Molecules Against IgE

The discovery of IgE back in 1966 was a watershed event in allergy history. Allergists hoped that it would unlock the door to both better diagnosis and targeted treatment. Unfortunately, it did not live up to the billing. The presence of allergen-specific IgE (sIgE) in the blood does not mean that you will react to that allergen. It must be attached to effector cells via high-affinity receptors. When it is floating in the blood, which is what most allergy blood tests actually measure, it is just a fuse without a bomb.

Section 4.2.2.4 of the 2010 NIAID Food Allergy Guidelines reads:

> *The (expert panel) recommends sIgE tests for identifying foods that potentially provoke IgE-mediated food-induced allergic reactions, but alone these tests are not diagnostic of FA....The presence of sIgE reflects allergic sensitization and not necessarily clinical allergy. Several studies comparing the quantity of sIgE to oral food challenges have reported that the greater the levels of sIgE, the higher the probability that ingestion of the food will lead to an allergic reaction. However, the predictive values varied from one study to another. This inconsistency may be due to multiple factors, such as patients' ages, duration of food allergen avoidance at the time of testing, selection of patients, and clinical disorders of patients being studied.*
>
> *Undetectable sIgE levels occasionally occur in patients with IgE-mediated FA. Therefore, in cases where the history is highly suggestive, further evaluation (for example, physician-supervised oral food challenge) is necessary before telling a patient that he or she is not allergic to a suspected food and may ingest it.[2]*

---

[2] "Guidelines for the diagnosis and management of food allergy in the United States: Report of the NIAID-sponsored expert panel," *Journal of Allergy and Clinical Immunology* December 2010; 126(6): 1105–1118.

Once a diagnosis of food allergy has been made on the basis of a clinical history of a reaction supported by judicious use of IgE levels and other testing, patients, parents, and their physicians continue to rely on IgE testing to monitor severity and look for downward trends and hope that an allergy may be outgrown. Since there has been no treatment for food allergy, this is often an exercise in wishful thinking.

Watching the numbers is a factor in Dr. Li's practice, too. Treating food allergies together with recalcitrant eczema and difficult-to-control asthma usually produces visible results and improves quality of life, whereas treating food allergies alone is harder to monitor, and parents watch IgE levels the way farmers watch weather reports during a drought.

Recognizing the importance of IgE as a "mother marker", i.e., a clinical benchmark that parents can focus on during "invisible" treatment; in 2013, Dr. Li and her team undertook an experiment to see if IgE production could be suppressed directly without any damage to the immune system.

TCM Therapy Effect on Peanut Specific IgE levels >100 KU/L (p7-8)

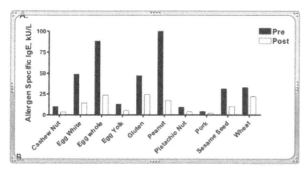

➤Fig shows peanut-specific IgE > 100 KU/L before TCM in a 3 y/o boy.
➤His IgE level was reduced by 93% gradually over a 3-year course of TCM treatment.

There had been previous efforts at attacking IgE directly, notably "anti-IgE" drugs. The initial anti-IgE drug, TNX-901, mothballed when the company that created it was acquired by the maker of the monoclonal antibody omalizumab (Xolair). This powerful drug is used primarily for severe asthma, but has been used in research to accompany oral immunotherapy for food allergies. It is expensive, sometimes painful, produces frequent adverse reactions, and must be administered by specialists.

Dr. Li's team set out to investigate the direct effects on IgE production of FAHF-2, and the refined, butanol-extracted version B-FAHF-2. Butanol extraction is used to separate the active, non-polar ingredients from the inert components of the full version. Finally, they set out to identify active components in individual herbs and test their effects using *in vitro* B-cell lines and human peripheral blood mononuclear cells (PBMCs) from food-allergic patients.[3]

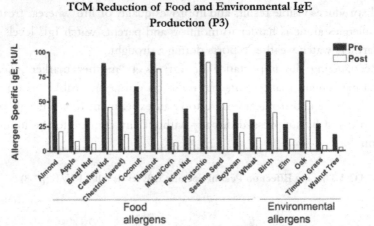

TCM Reduction of Food and Environmental IgE Production (P3)

Patient 3 as in table 1 (9 y/o): IgE Levels Before & After TCM. Patient 3 showed poly-sensitization to multiple foods & environmental allergens. Bar graph shows representative IgE levels that were >15kU/L before TCM, which were reduced after 7 months of TCM: almond from 55.8 to 19.9, cashew from 89.00 to 44.5, coconut from 65.3 to 37, hazelnut from >100 to 83.3, pecan nut from 42.7, pistachio from >100 to 89, sesame from >100 to 48.1, birch from >100 to 38.5, oak from >100 to 50.4. Total IgE decreased from 1,953 to 881.

Individual compounds were isolated and identified using column chromatography, liquid chromatographic mass spectrometry, and nuclear magnetic resonance techniques. Once isolated, the team first tested the compounds on U266 cells, which are a B cell line that is easily grown in the

[3] Nan Yang, PhD; Julie Wang, MD; Changda Liu, PhD; Ying Song, MD; Shuwei Zhang, PhD; Jiachen Zi, PhD; Jixun Zhan, PhD; Madhan Masilamani, PhD; Amanda Cox, MD; Anna Nowak-Wegrzyn, MD; Hugh Sampson, MD; and Xiu-Min Li, MD, MS, "Berberine and limonin suppress IgE production by human B cells and peripheral blood mononuclear cells from food-allergic patients," *Annals of Allergy, Asthma and Immunology* 2014; 113(5): 556–564.e4.

lab. This is a good first step because B cells are responsible for manufacturing and secreting antibodies such as IgE. Compounds were also tested and verified using human peripheral blood mononuclear cells (PBMCs) from blood samples obtained from 20 boys and 5 girls with food allergy, ages 6–17. All children had physician-documented histories of allergic reactions to peanut and/or tree nut and/or fish with a positive skin test result and/or food allergen specific IgE level for peanut, tree nut or fish specific IgE above 0.7 kU/L.

The researchers studied various biochemical markers with the hope that all or some of these could point the way to being able to measure progress, including transcript expression, phosphorylated IkBa levels, mRNA expression of signal transducer and activator of transcription-3. T-box transcription factor TBX21, interferon-g, forkhead box P3, GATA-binding protein 3, interleukin-10, and interleukin-5 were also analyzed using real-time polymerase chain reaction.

To evaluate the effects of FAHF-2 on IgE production, U266 cells were incubated with FAHF-2 at different concentrations. FAHF-2 inhibited IgE production with higher dosages significantly more effectively than lower ones. At the highest concentration (500 mg/mL), inhibition reached 78.1%.

The butanol version, B-FAHF-2, was also tested on U266 cells at concentrations of 0, 7.5, 15, 30, 60, and 120 mg/mL, which were equivalent to that of FAHF-2 based on yield value from previous experiments. B-FAHF-2 also inhibited IgE production by U266 cells in a dose-dependent manner. Suppression of IgE by B-FAHF-2 reached statistical significance at 30, 60, and 120 mg/mL ($P < .001$) and maximally inhibited IgE production (92.0%) at the highest concentration (120 mg/mL), which indicated that B-FAHF-2 achieves the same inhibitory level at a dose 9.2-fold lower than for FAHF-2 (34.44 vs 313.6 mg/mL). Trypan blue exclusion assays showed that neither FAHF-2 and B-FAHF-2 had harmful effects on cell viability at the concentrations used.

These data show that B-FAHF-2, comprised of only the less-polar components found in the original FAHF-2, is more potent than FAHF-2 at inhibiting IgE production. This finding is consistent with high-performance liquid chromatography (HPLC) fingerprint features of B-FAHF- 2 and FAHF-2. Although 36 peaks were detected in FAHF-2 and B-FAHF-2, B-FAHF-2 showed greater intensity for most less-polar and nonpolar peaks even at an approximately 5-fold lower HPLC loading concentration (40 mg/mL) than FAHF-2 (198 mg/mL).

Philodendron chinensis aqueous extracts were further isolated and fractionated, and 2 compounds, DMF-A1 (compound 1) and DMF-C1 (compound 2), were purified. These two compounds were isolated for having the greatest potential effect on IgE — berberine and limonin. (For those who despise industrial food processing: While ultimately found to be the less potent of the two, limonin is described in the paper as a natural component of citrus fruit that lends a slightly sour note. According to the authors, limonin is removed from juice to make it sweeter.)[4]

Using berberine or limonin at different concentrations, the team studied their bioactivity levels *in vitro* on U266 cells. Berberine inhibited IgE production in a dose-dependent manner, reaching 94.6% inhibition at 20 mg/mL. Limonin showed a mild decrease of IgE production by U266 cells. The greatest inhibitory effect of limonin was 35.1%, observed at a concentration of 20 mg/mL (P < .01). Unlike berberine, no dose-dependent effect was observed for limonin. Cell viability assays showed no toxicity at any concentration tested.

The lack of cytotoxicity sparked a unique avenue of inquiry. We know that many good drugs have bad side effects. For example, systemic steroids treat allergic inflammation but make us vulnerable to other infections. Because berberine suppressed IgE production without killing any cells, the team set out to find out how it switched the cell's protein manufacturing machinery on and off. Bellanti *et al.*[5] describe "a cascading series of enzymatic responses" they call the "Three T's" — Transduction, Transcription, and Translation. First, the cell must receive a signal and "transduce" the appropriate cellular response — i.e., change one kind of message into another. In this case, the cells were transducing a signal coming from berberine. Next, transcription takes place when particular regions of DNA generate messenger RNA containing the "'blueprint' for the protein in the next step." The final step is translation, when the messenger RNA intermediate code is made into a protein product, such as further regulatory

[4] *Ibid.*

[5] Joseph A. Bellanti, MD, *Immunology IV Clinical Applications in Health and Disease* 2012; I Care Press, Bethesda, Maryland, p. 181.

proteins broadly called transcription factors or IgE antibodies themselves.

Dr. Li says when this goes wrong, it is like front line officers getting bad orders from their commanders. She and her co-authors wrote,

Although there are no direct studies on whether and how berberine suppresses IgE synthesis, some studies have shown that berberine suppresses NF-kB signaling pathways, which is associated with its anti-cancer, anti-inflammatory, and anti-diabetic actions.

The experiments showed that berberine increased the production, i.e., expression, of several transcription factors, STAT3, Foxp3, and T-bet. When these transcription factors have weak expression levels, they are linked to increased IgE production. Limonin was therapeutic, but all in all, it was not as potent as berberine by these measures.

What does this mean to food-allergy patients? Possibly a yardstick for measuring progress during a long course of therapy. Short-term suppression of the allergic response does not mean that an allergy is cured. Dr. Li hopes that her therapy will work its way upstream to the "transduction" stage, to the memory cells that continue to recognize a harmless allergen as an enemy. No more bad orders from the generals.

Long term-treatment may lead to Dr. Li's vision of retraining the immune system. As she put it in the previous book, we want to turn bad boys into good boys. At the same time we want to avoid turning good girls bad.

Predicting a Reaction

Because the accustomed blood and skin tests are flawed tools for diagnosing food allergies with a high degree of accuracy, allergists and food allergy patients everywhere are anxious for something more accurate without the anxiety and risk that accompany a food challenge. Component testing[6] — a more refined blood IgE test — can show whether the patient is sensitized to particular parts of a protein associated with more or less severe reactions, but it is not definitive.

---

[6] These tests look at which parts of the protein the patient is reactive to; some components are associated with anaphylaxis and some with lesser reactions.

The basophil activation test (BAT) has attracted a great deal of attention for its potential to show a reaction safely outside the patient's body — a kind of controlled detonation on a desert test range.

Dr. Li's team explored the possibility that the BAT could stand in for a food challenge in a paper called "Correlations between Basophil Activation, Allergen-specific IgE with Outcome and Severity of Oral Food Challenges".[7]

The basophil is one of two "effector cells" that carry out an allergic reaction. The mast cell, which is better known, is embedded in tissue in various parts of the body that are regularly exposed to the wider environment — the skin, airways, lungs, and digestive tract. It bristles with IgE antibodies attached to high-affinity receptors and when the allergic antigen presents itself, it in effect completes a circuit and the cell degranulates, releasing the "toxic soup" of mediators meant to fight the antigen.

Unlike the mast cell, the basophil circulates in the blood allowing it to reinforce the first wave of reaction. It is responsible for late-phase allergic reactions. Unlike mast cells, which would have to be dug out of tissue to test, the basophil can be extracted from a blood sample and exposed to an allergen to see whether it will react or not.

Patients aged 12 through 45 years old with a convincing history of allergy to peanut, tree nut, sesame, fish, or shrimp undergoing DBPCFCs as part of screening for enrollment in the FAHF-2 clinical trial were included in this study. Skin prick tests, allergen-specific IgE, and component tests were done to see which would correlate with a true clinical reaction as determined by the DBPCFCs.

Eventually 58 of 66 subjects reacted to the actual food challenge.

To investigate whether the BAT could distinguish subjects with both positive and negative DBPCFC reactions, three concentrations were used for each allergen. In this study, the BAT proved the best predictor of clinical reactivity.

When word of this study circulated, many food allergy parents inquired, if a blood test could indeed predict the outcome of a food challenge, where

[7] "Correlations between basophil activation, allergen-specific IgE with outcome and severity of oral food challenges," Ying Song, MD; Julie Wang, MD; Nicole Leung, BS; Li Xin Wang, MD, PhD; Lauren Lisann, BS; Scott H. Sicherer, MD; Amy M. Scurlock, MD; Robbie Pesek, MD; Tamara T. Perry, MD; Stacie M. Jones, MD; Xiu-Min Li, MD, MS, *Annals of Allergy, Asthma and Immunology* 2015; 114: 319e326.

could they get it? I had to explain that not only is it expensive, it is currently wildly impractical for routine clinical use. Unlike IgE tests, the blood must be drawn at the site where the test will be performed. It is in effect a live reaction. Each potential allergen must be tested individually, not done with an array of allergens. This makes it inappropriate for your corner allergist. Nor is it coded for insurance reimbursement. However, as interest grows in this technique, it is conceivable that it will be added to the services at regional food allergy centers, as envisioned by Food Allergy Research and Education (FARE), which, in its various incarnations, has funded major work in the field.

"Tolerance in a Test Tube"

If the BAT is limited as a diagnostic, routine use for measuring progress toward outgrowing a food allergy would seem even more impractical. The trajectories of food allergies are pretty well studied. Guideline 3.1 reads,

> Most children with FA eventually will tolerate milk, egg, soy, and wheat; far fewer will eventually tolerate tree nuts and peanut. The time course of FA resolution in children varies by food and may occur as late as the teenage years. A high initial level of sIgE against a food is associated with a lower rate of resolution of clinical allergy over time.

Higher initial numbers and severity of skin-prick tests are associated with persistent allergy.

Because there has never been a cure for food allergies and immunotherapy is largely experimental, incentives to measure patient progress during therapy have been absent. Most patients have managed the problem by avoiding the foods and preparing for emergencies while waiting for nature to take its course. Allergen-specific IgE levels in the blood may rise and fall. Food challenges are the truest test, but they are not suitable for periodic use, and they are so anxiety provoking that many people do not try them even after their allergist recommends it. If, however, a reasonably expeditious long-term treatment could be found, tools to show "tolerance in a test tube" would be warranted.

This possibility was suggested by laboratory experience. Dr. Li says,

> *When we've taken blood to look at the cells, for example, and mixed it with peanut protein — two nanograms — a very low dosage. Before treatment the cells produce*

60–90% activation, meaning 60–90% of the cells release histamine. This shows that the patient is very sensitive. Then after treatment, we've done the same blood sample mixed with two nanograms of peanut protein, and seen 20% of the basophil cells release histamine. From this we know that tolerance has increased (non-allergic people also have basophil activation, about 10–20%). So that gives us a quantitative measurement.

In 2014, with the BAT paper in the works, and with B-FAHF-2 showing such promise, Dr. Li and her team began to plot a study to use it as a biomarker for response to treatment. The working title is "Practice-Based Bio-Marker Study using Traditional Chinese Medicine to Prove Real Life Effects on Patients with Poly-Allergen Sensitization."[8]

As explained in a post published[9] on the website (which I edit), Dr. Li and two co-investigators, both allopathic allergists, wrote:

> The results to date [with B-FAHF-2] are sufficiently encouraging to treat patients in a practice-based study and see if we can measure progress by examining changes in the blood chemistry. The first cohort of approximately 50 patients who meet study criteria will be treated through our combined efforts.
>
> We will be looking at several bio-markers — chemical indicators that correspond to changes in immune activity.

In addition to the BAT, another is DNA methylation by the Th1 and Th2 cells.

> DNA methylation determines "gene expression" — turning on and off cellular secretion of certain cytokines (small proteins that help regulate the immune response). In a healthy immune system, Th1 cells dominate, helping fight infectious disease. In an allergic individual, Th2 cells, which are normally associated with fighting invasive parasites, are too powerful, and they attack proteins in things like pollens and foods. We are going to study two markers: (1) IFN-γ, the principal Th1 effector cytokine, which plays a crucial

---

[8] Notably, the first phase of this study was "crowd funded" by individuals.
[9] http://www.asthmaallergieschildren.com. First posted on December 4, 2014.

role in counteracting and suppressing Th2 responses of allergic diseases. It is deficient in food allergic patients; (2) RANTES (CCL5), which is highly secreted in food allergy patients and plays an important role in recruiting basophils, eosinophils, and T cells into the inflammatory sites.

This study will differ in significant ways from the normal protocols. As a "proof of concept," it will lay the groundwork for much larger research in years to come. This is a practice-based study. Subjects will not undergo food challenges at baseline. Rather, they will be rigorously screened by the participating allopathic physicians to ensure they all meet the criteria for serious food allergies. There will be no placebo controls. Everyone will receive TCM treatment, which will include not only B-FAHF-2, but, because many patients will have co-morbid eczema and asthma, other treatments as well. There will be an observational control group in the form of *in vitro* blood taken from patients with poly-allergen sensitization who have never received TCM or other treatments beyond a medically restricted diet. These untreated samples will undergo the same tests of the treated blood for comparison.

As Dr. Li says,

> *There are three requirements for the individuals in the study. They have to have a history of reactions and their peanut specific IgE has to be over 100. Or if the peanut IgE is not over one hundred, but I look at the two-year IgE figures and see it's very high and increasing, those patients can also qualify. The third group will be made up of people who have a history and very frequent reactions. You know sometimes children are so sensitive, they don't even have to eat the offending food, they just smell it or touch it and they have a reaction. They will also qualify. This is a patient friendly protocol.*

There will be three courses of treatment, each lasting a year.

> *I believe we'll see changes in biomarkers in the first year for some, such as reduced basophil activity, but for others it may take two or three years. Maybe someone after one year will see effects. If the IgE is more than 100, in one or two years you'll start to see it drop — but it may not drop to the level where it's so low that they can go for a challenge. Other biomarkers will help to monitor progress. You have to separate when the effects*

are first visible and there is tolerance from the child "outgrowing" the allergy, which may take longer.

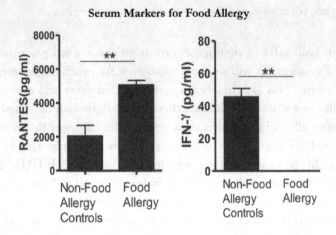

Eventually, if patients' immunological responses (IgE levels, basophil activation and T cell epigenetic status) are dramatically improved by treatment compared to baseline, and if the family is interested in introducing certain foods, the doctors will determine clinical tolerability using standard allergy protocols, or perhaps using newer tools now in development that are considered highly predictive of the results of a food challenge. For example, an algorithm by Irish and British researchers called the Cork-Southampton Food Challenge Outcome Calculator, which combines skin prick test responses, serum specific IgE levels, total IgE levels minus serum-specific IgE levels, symptoms, sex, and age seems to predict the outcome of oral food challenge with a high degree of accuracy, both positive and negative.[10]

The authors write:

> Unlike other studies, in which subjects usually have a narrow set of allergic conditions at baseline, this one is more like the "real world" of food

---

[10]Audrey Dunn Galvin, PhD; L.M. Segal, MD; Ann Clarke, MD, MSc, FRCP; Reza Alizadehfar, MD; Jonathan O'B.Hourihane, PhD Med, MB, MRCPI, FRCPCH, "Validation of the Cork-Southampton food challenge outcome calculator in a Canadian sample," *Journal of Allergy and Clinical Immunology* January 2013; 131(1): 230–232.

allergic patients. Those with severe food allergies often have other allergic diseases, and they can take part in this research, where in other studies they might be excluded. This study is also suitable for children with multiple food allergies who have histories of severe reactions. It is patient friendly and cost effective. The data will be important for designing a controlled, prospective study and for NIH funding application in the future. If successful, this protocol can be adopted by other allergists in their practices. Also, because TCM is inherently an individualized approach to medicine, other herbal drugs, as well as acupuncture and acupressure, may be used for different patients depending on their other conditions. This will not compromise the integrity of the biomarker data.

Among many things that distinguish Dr. Li's work from other researchers is the conduct of world-class research in parallel with a clinical practice. The science informs the practice, which informs the science.

We are pioneers. It's not perfect yet. There are lots of knowledge gaps. That's why in addition to continuing double blind placebo controlled trials, we will also conduct practice-based evidence (PBE) studies, which is more cost effective and will help design an even better trial in the near future.

Practice-based evidence studies that use existing treatment, are an alternative to randomized controlled trials, and well suited to determine what works best for specific patient types in day-to-day clinical practice. They provide a holistic picture of patients, treatments, and outcomes seen in real-world clinical settings. They can uncover better practices more quickly than randomized trials, while achieving many of the same advantages. TCM is inherently an individualized approach using Chinese herbal medicines as well as acupuncture and acupressure; PBE studies are well suited to define what TCM therapies will be the best for the specific group of patients with food allergies.

Thus, when the dosing requirements of FAHF-2 ran headlong into the realities of human behavior, there was a relentless push to find a more concentrated version.

In her introduction to this book, Dr. Li displays that special triad of perspectives — scientist, healer, and mother — that impels her forward. They are ever present. She says,

I've really learned a lot from mothers. I started to work on my case reports because a mother said, "You have so many good results, why don't you publish them? Do a small

study not a big trial study and publish it." I've got medical students helping me organize the data. We don't always know which element is essential to clinical efficacy. We can find out, as in the berberine-limonin study, but sometimes we can see results, and it's important to show that, too.

A prime example is this case study of three patients whose lives were fractured by their food allergies.

Three Cases of Frequent Severe Food Anaphylaxis

Much of the time, most patients who suffer from anaphylactic food allergies are symptom free. They dutifully avoid their allergens and carry their emergency epinephrine. They walk a fine line, but at least their feet are on the ground, and they can lead rewarding lives.

However, there are some for whom day-to-day existence is closer to a tightrope. In 2014, Dr. Li and several co-authors compiled three cases of frequent severe food anaphylaxis (FSFA), published in an article called "Successful Prevention of Extremely Frequent and Severe Food Anaphylaxis in Three Children by Combined Traditional Chinese Medicine Therapy".[11]

This article was significant for many reasons, one of which is that it is a prototype for more examples of her publication of "practice based evidence." Dr. Li's approximately 100 publications are dominated by research, but as the practice grows, so do the results. In practice, she employs versions of the registered investigational drugs but she is not bound by the necessity for uniform treatment or blinding that come with a clinical trial. Even the practice-based research, which will be discussed later, can employ a range of tools.

The inclusion criteria for the three patients were: physician (allergist) diagnosed severe food allergy (as documented by physician-determined history of allergic reactions to food allergen, a positive skin test result and/or elevated food allergen specific IgE level), clinical reactions that became

---

[11] Lauren Lisann, Ying Song, Julie Wang, Paul Ehrlich, Anne Maitland and Xiu-Min Li, "Successful prevention of extremely frequent and severe food anaphylaxis in three children by combined traditional Chinese medicine therapy," *Allergy, Asthma and Clinical Immunology* 2014; 10(66), DOI:10.1186/s13223-014-0066-5.

worse over time prior to TCM treatment, and experienced FSFA including multiple life-threatening episodes (>10 reactions and >2 epinephrine uses in the three months prior to starting TCM therapy), adherence to the TCM regimen, and had completed at least six months of TCM therapy. Concurrent use of omalizumab was excluded.

TCM therapy consisted of Modified *Pruni Mume* Formula (Remedy A), *Fructus Jujubae* Formula (Remedy B), a *Phellodendron chinensis* (*P. chinesis*) containing herbal bath additive (Remedy C), and herbal cream (Remedy D). Remedies A and B were used as dietary supplements. Use of additional herbs is noted in each case discussion when applicable. Acupuncture/acupressure was also administered during TCM clinic visits.

Patient 1 was a 13-year-old female who had been diagnosed with milk allergy at three months of age after an ER visit due to anaphylaxis (widespread hives, vomiting and difficulty breathing) immediately following ingestion of cow-milk-based formula. The frequency and severity of her reactions worsened over time. Despite a dairy restricted diet, during the two-year period prior to starting TCM she averaged 50 reactions/year). Fifty events in all required prednisone and epinephrine, 40 required ER visits, and 3 intensive care unit (ICU) admissions. In the three months before TCM, her reactions became even more severe; five of ten events required epinephrine and ER visits. Symptoms included hives, rash, lip swelling, throat tightness, wheezing, stomach pain, headache, weakness, dizziness, syncope, hypoxia, and drop in blood pressure. Reactions were triggered by inhalation and contact in addition to accidental ingestion. Anaphylaxis events were so frequent and severe that she was unable to attend school in the four months prior to her first TCM visit. She also complained of chronic stomach discomfort. Her milk-protein specific IgE levels were elevated at 37.3 kU/L but she had no skin-prick tests because of severe reactions from skin contact.

She was prescribed all four TCM remedies. Since her reactions often began with throat tightness or pain, *Fructus Arctii Lappae*, which has been traditionally used for throat ailments, was added. Acupuncture was also performed at each visit. She tolerated the medicine very well and after approximately three months no longer complained of stomach discomfort. Follow-up visits took place every 3–6 months, for a total of eight follow-up visits. Her FSFA slightly improved after six months of TCM and greatly improved after 1½ years of TCM, and she went back to school. After two years, reactions were reduced by 90%. None required epinephrine, or ER visits. Symptom severity was reduced by 56%. She was able to work a summer job as a lifeguard, and she and her father no longer feared flying to New York for her two-year TCM visit. She experienced no reactions during the final six months. Her baseline milk specific IgE level of 37.3 kU/L has declined to 19.0 kU/L. She is continuing TCM therapy with a new goal of maintaining the beneficial effect and to possibly become tolerant to milk allergens.

Patient 2 was a 16-year-old female diagnosed with severe nut allergy at age 13 after an ER visit for anaphylaxis triggered by eating in a Thai restaurant, exhibited as widespread hives, lip swelling and vomiting, followed by throat tightness and difficulty breathing. Despite abstaining from nuts and daily diphenhydramine and cetirizine during the two years prior to starting TCM, she experienced 30 severe reactions requiring 34 epinephrine and 30 additional diphenhydramine doses, and 10 ER admissions. One episode required four epinephrine doses prior to emergency hospital admission following helicopter transport. She was most sensitive to almonds, and vomited and developed widespread hives after skin prick testing with almond two years prior to TCM. During the year prior to TCM, her reactions progressed much more rapidly from hives and vomiting to hypoxia and circulatory collapse. She was severely sensitive to trace nut inhalation and contact. She missed approximately 50% of school days and had to withdraw from school sports. She developed anxiety/depression and was on antidepressants. Her mother (an ER physician) arranged numerous consultations with allergists. They were subsequently told that there was nothing more to be done, and there was nothing on the horizon that would help her severe nut anaphylaxis. After the mother read publications showing that TCM herbal medicines abolished food anaphylaxis in murine models, they sought similar therapy.

This patient followed the same initial protocol as Patient 1. However, unlike Patient 1, she responded relatively quickly, experiencing only one reaction during the first three months of treatment (moderate hives, face swelling, and throat pain, but no gastrointestinal symptoms, wheezing, cardiovascular, or neurological symptoms). She maintained intake of ten pills of Remedy A (twice daily). Her anxiety also dramatically improved and she discontinued antidepressants after two months of TCM. After 4–6 months of TCM, she experienced two mild reactions. The first included mild hives, rash, and lip swelling only, and was treated with antihistamines. The second reaction consisted of a few hives. After six months, she discontinued daily antihistamine use. She experienced no reactions during months 10–12 of treatment. Since she lives in another country, her mother had monthly phone consultations for the first two months, and then every 2–3 months plus email communication until completing one year of TCM therapy, at which time she passed a nut challenge. The tentative 12-month visit was cancelled. Her mother continued to communicate by emails up to six months after challenge. During this period she accidentally consumed nut-containing pastry and experienced no allergic reaction. She subsequently passed challenges with almond and mixed nuts and now eats them whenever she wants.

Patient 3 was a 9-year-old male with severe tree nut and fruit allergies who began TCM therapy in June 2013 with the goal of reducing the frequency of his reactions. He was diagnosed with nut allergy at age 7 after an ER visit due to anaphylaxis (projectile vomiting, inability to move his legs due to cramps, throat closed, diffuse hives and breathing difficulty) after ingesting chocolate containing mixed nuts. Despite an all-nut-restricted diet, his reactions became more frequent and severe. He also developed reactions to additional foods, including coconut, sesame seed, certain fruits and wheat, which he had previously tolerated. Reactions were triggered by inhalation and contact as well as accidental ingestion of trace amounts of offending foods. During the prior two-year period he experienced approximately 400 reactions (every few days and at times daily, averaging 200 reactions per year) while on daily levocetirizine. His allergist added daily fexofenadine because levocetirizine alone failed to reduce the number or severity of reactions during the prior six months. However, his frequent reactions did not decrease. His most common reactions included widespread itching, diffuse hives, swollen tongue, projectile vomiting, and throat tightness. The most severe reactions included wheezing, hypoxia, muscle cramping, weakness, and increased heart rate. Five reactions required epinephrine and ER visits. He had positive skin test results to almond, pistachio, sesame, peanut, soybean, coconut, apple and wheat in the six months prior to TCM. Extensive serum IgE testing ordered by his primary allergist two years and one month prior to his initial TCM visit revealed that he was poly-sensitized to multiple food and environmental allergens. His IgE levels to 65 food and environmental allergens were elevated. Seventeen were above 17.6 KU/L (classified as very high), 13 of these were to food allergens. He had a history of reactions to all 13 foods, but was most sensitive to almonds. He also complained of chronic stomach discomfort and headaches, and developed a sleep disorder approximately six months before beginning TCM treatment.

This patient underwent the same regimen as the first two patients. However, the maximum dose of Remedy A was 8 pills, twice a day (adjusted based on his age, approximately 1/3 of full dose). He also received monthly acupuncture. Frequency and severity of his reactions fell 50% during the first three months of TCM (from 20 reactions per month at baseline to 10). During the 4–6 months treatment period, he experienced only two mild reactions. He has discontinued fexofenadine. After seven months of TCM, he also discontinued levocetirizine, and he has experienced only one mild reaction treated with diphenhydramine. His overall symptom score declined from 24 to 1. All 17 foods and environmental allergen-specific IgE levels, previously above 17.6 kU/L, were reduced. Liver and kidney function test results were all within the normal range before and after TCM. In addition, after the first three months of treatment, he no longer experienced stomach discomfort, headaches, or disordered sleep. He reached his primary goal, and is continuing TCM therapy to maintain the efficacy and perhaps to induce tolerance to some of the foods.

The cases in this paper are significant for many reasons, not least of which is the profound relief to the patients and their families, who spent each day for years with the sword of anaphylaxis hanging over their heads. It also tackles head on the cases where contact and inhalation are the precipitating events. Patient reports of anaphylaxis via the air and contact are so rare that many allergists dismiss them altogether, but they were quite real to these patients, and to Dr. Li.

Treating Digestion

Food allergens that make it through the caldron of enzymes and acids on their way to the duodenum, the first portion of the small intestine, where they can be absorbed into the blood stream are rugged things. They are often storage proteins, built by nature to survive dormancy and winter and nourish the next generation of peanuts or tree nuts as they germinate. The protein components that are most likely to trigger anaphylaxis, such as Arah1, 2, and 3 in peanuts, are heat stabile and they stand up better to the chemical assault of the gastrointestinal tract than heat labile proteins like Arah8, which is an environmental allergen akin to birch pollen. These birch pollen allergens are common in many fruits and vegetables, as well as trees and flowers, but they generally result at most in symptoms referred to as oral allergy syndrome (OAS). They are in effect sinus allergies delivered by food and degraded after they are swallowed. Uncomfortable but generally not dangerous. It is those harder storage proteins that cause most of the worry.

According to Dr. Li,

One particular group of patients are children who when they were little, only had a few allergies. But as they grow, they acquire more and more food allergies. They develop environmental allergies as well. For them, I see that the digestive system is not functioning properly — in addition to the immune system and IgE. For these patients, I've begun to deepen the treatment with great TCM principles — not simply using a formula that matches the symptoms.

I discussed this problem with Dr. Li on and off for a few years. Among the factors we have talked about are the depleted microbiome from antibiotics and Caesarian birth, but also the sweetness of refined Western diets, which also complicates treatment. American children have a tough time tolerating bitter herbal treatments, which are second nature to most Chinese kids.

But it is the chemistry of digestion that concerns her most, the ability to break down routine proteins into units that nourish the body, not threaten it.

Sometimes we forget the physiological function of digestion. So that's why I developed a treatment called digestion tea. To help the kids rebuild their GI system. That's really a TCM concept. They have this concept that they focus for children on enhancing the GI system.

What makes these little digestive systems allergy prone? Eva Untersmayr, MD, PhD, Head of the Gastrointestinal Immunology research at the Medical

University of Vienna, wrote an article for my website,[12] which recapitulated her previously published peer-reviewed papers. She said,

> Under normal conditions, high acidity–low pH is responsible for activating the main enzyme for fragmenting proteins in the stomach. The partially digested acidic food — called chyme — then arrives in the upper part of the small intestine, the duodenum, triggering the release of enzymes from the pancreas.
>
> However, in situations of high pH–low acid production in the stomach, also called hypoacidity, these enzymes do not become activated. Gastric hypoacidity is not a rare condition. It is found both in newborns and infants in the first two years of life, and also in older patients. For small children, this leaves a window of opportunity for sensitization to complex proteins. For their part, more than half of patients older than 60 have reduced gastric acid production, which may account for many complaints from grandparents after a holiday dinner, or general loss of appetite as food just "sits there" instead of passing through comfortably.

Dr. Untersmayr has also studied the phenomenon of otherwise healthy adults becoming allergic to particular foods while under treatment for heartburn with antacids, protein pump inhibitors, and other medicines.

Standard allergy treatment seems to ignore the connection between immunity and digestion, which seems so obvious in Dr. Li's approach. It is particularly disturbing because gastric distress is a frequent side effect of oral immunotherapy (OIT), the food allergy treatment that is likely to become the first mainstream therapy for food allergies. Private practitioners who are already doing OIT are reported to resort to reflux treatments for their patients who are having trouble swallowing their daily doses rather than abandon their immunotherapy, when this may be counterproductive. Dr. Untersmayr says,

> I am concerned at anecdotal reports of antacid use to suppress vomiting during oral immunotherapy. I feel that because the concomitant use of antacids with ingestion of allergenic proteins may induce food allergy to begin with, their regular use with proven allergens could make digestive systems even more vulnerable.

---

[12] http://asthmaallergieschildren.com/2013/08/23/protect-your-digestion-the-first-line-of-defense-against-food-allergies/

Because of the link between OIT and gastric symptoms, Dr. Li has added two categories to her list of conditions treated — "Oral Immunotherapy (OIT) for food allergy patients in both clinical trials and private (non-FDA-approved) treatment who have been forced to drop out because of frequent gastric distress and other adverse reactions, " as well as "OIT patients in private clinics with GI symptoms who are persisting with treatment but seeking relief."

Postscript

Dr. Li's team has experimented with an additional solvent for refining the herbal formula. The early data show great promise for production efficiency and medical efficacy.

Chapter

2

ASTHMA

There's one particular ailment, though, for which I've always been singled out, so to speak. I see no reason to call it by its Greek name, difficulty in breathing being a perfectly good way of describing it. Its onslaught is of very brief duration — like a squall, it is generally over within the hour. One could hardly, after all, expect anyone to keep on drawing his last breath for long, could one? I have suffered every kind of unpleasant or dangerous physical complaint, but none is worse than this. Not surprising, for anything else is just an illness, while this is gasping out your life-breath. That is why doctors call it a "rehearsal for death", since eventually the breath does what it has often been trying to do (Lucius Annaeus Seneca, 4 BC–65 AD).[13]

Asthma is clearly not a new disease. According to the World Allergy Organization 2011 White Book, some 300 million people suffer from it worldwide and it contributes to the deaths of 250,000 people annually. In the United States, 9.3% of children and 8% of adults have asthma. Economic costs to the United States approach $60 billion each year in treatment, 10.5 million missed days of school, and 14.2 million missed days of work. About nine people die from asthma every day, well over 3,000 each year.

---

[13] From *Asthma: The Biography* by Mark Jackson. It should be noted that asthma played no part in Seneca's death, which was by his own hand for conspiring against Emperor Nero.

That is more than the entire death toll from allergic anaphylaxis for a 12-year period, most of them from medication allergies, followed by insect stings, and finally food allergies.[14] Poorly controlled asthma can have very serious consequences for food allergy patients with no previous history of respiratory reactions.

One way of looking at respiratory anaphylaxis is as an asthma attack set off by a trigger presented to the lungs via the blood instead of inhaled, such as pollen or chemical particulates. Uncontrolled asthma puts the patient at risk of death, but body counts are not the only important measure. There is also the danger of "airway remodeling" — structural changes that significantly impair normal lung function. While many types of lung structures may be "remodeled," one key example involves the lungs' airway smooth muscles (ASMs) — a loss of elasticity from what we might call the Arnold Schwarzenegger effect. With normal breathing, ASMs get the right amount of exercise to stay toned. However, when they are abnormally stressed because of allergic reactions, cold air, or dryness, resulting in bronchoconstriction, the muscles get what amounts to an extra heavy workout. They thicken and lose the flexibility they need for normal breathing. Lungs exchange gasses less efficiently than they should. Day-to-day, airway remodeling brings with it a diminished quality of life — for children, disordered sleep, half-hearted play, poor athleticism, and inattentiveness at school; for adults, missed days of work or "presenteeism" — a word that describes lack of productivity at a job because of illness and sleep deprivation.

Asthma is a personal issue for me. When I was 12, having suffered from severe environmental allergies for years, I got a summer job with a friend working in a commercial nursery owned by a local family. On very hot, humid days, we ducked frequently into the greenhouse and stuck our heads into the fine mist sprayed over the plants several times an hour. Between the allergens emitted by the plants, the agricultural chemicals, and the intermittent heating and cooling, I started to struggle with my breathing, which made an accordion noise as I tried to speak.

---

[14]Elina Jerschow, MD, MSc; Robert Y. Lin, MD, MSc; Moira M. Scaperotti, BS; Aileen P. McGinn, PhD, "Fatal anaphylaxis in the United States, 1999–2010: Temporal patterns and demographic associations," *Journal of Allergy and Clinical Immunology* December 2014; 134(6): 1318–1328.e.

My middle child also had some allergies, but no history of asthma until one July when I had a sudden call with the news that he was in the local hospital on a regimen of nebulizers and steroids. A combination of leaf mold and wood smoke from a campfire had triggered an attack. Both my son and I eventually benefited from courses of allergy shots, delivered over 30 years apart, of course. What has surprised me in my ongoing reading about the disease is how little progress there has been in curing asthma in the years in between my son's and my own exacerbations. As immunologist Dr. Arnold Levinson has pointed out, there had been no fundamental breakthrough in asthma treatment after the 1980 synthesis of inhaled corticosteroids (ICS) from a botanical source, diosgenin in yams, instead of from animal byproducts. A newer treatment, bronchothermoplasty, uses heat to burn away tissue in airways that have become "muscle bound" from years of bronchoconstriction. It is performed over three outpatient sessions and costs about $20,000.

While ICS remain the dominant treatment for controlling asthmatic inflammation, they, like powerful systemic steroids, have some serious side effects. Notably, they suppress the part of the endocrine system, called the hypothalamic-pituitary-adrenal axis, which assists the immune system's fight against viral and bacterial infection and produces cortisol, the body's own anti-inflammatory. Long-term steroid treatments also have serious implications for mood disorders, both anxiety and depression. These issues, as you will read, helped guide the research described in these pages.

Furthermore, we have also learned that asthma is not a single disease but a syndrome — a collection of symptoms. Many patients have "non-allergic asthma" and fail to respond to standard medications. It is also called steroid-resistant asthma, which does not bear further definition, except insofar as non-specialist physicians try to treat it with steroids anyway, so patients get all the side effects with none of the therapy.

Dr. Anthony Gagliardi has described the study of asthma as "the study of one patient." That is, diagnosis and treatment cannot be generalized since asthma is no longer considered a single disease. There are too many variables. The number of phenotypes — observed categories of disease that cannot be pinned down by testing — is long and growing by the week it seems: mild, moderate, severe; exercised-induced; cold-induced; baker's asthma (reacting to flour). In children: "transient infant wheezing which does not persist" and "persistent asthma." A common adult phenotype is aspirin/NSAID-sensitive asthma. Still another would be neutrophilic asthma (which does not respond to steroids) versus eosinophilic (which does) depending on the dominance of one white blood cell or the other. And so on. Approximately 83% of poorly controlled asthmatics have neutrophil-dominant sputum.[15]

Meanwhile, research dollars are poured into finding out what causes asthma with marginal and sometimes contradictory results. For example, a 2011 study in *Pediatrics* on a common drug said,

> [T]he evidence for a link between acetaminophen (aka paracetamol) and asthma is now strong enough for doctors to recommend that infants and children who have asthma (or are at risk for the disease) avoid acetaminophen.[16]

Four years later, the authors of an article in the *Journal of Allergy and Clinical Immunology*, found the link more tenuous:

> Adjustment for respiratory tract infections in early life substantially diminished associations between infant antipyretic [drugs for fever like Tylenol] use and early childhood asthma.[17]

A similar association between antibiotic use and asthma was addressed in a Swedish study published in 2014. Higher rates of asthma were seen among children who were being treated for respiratory infections than for other

---

[15] W.C. Moore, A.T. Hastie, X. Li, H. Li, W.W. Busse, N.N. Jarjour, S.E. Wenzel, S.P. Peters, D.A. Meyers, E.R. Bleecker, *et al.*, "Sputum neutrophil counts are associated with more severe asthma phenotypes using cluster analysis," *Journal of Allergy and Clinical Immunology* June 2014;133(6):1557–1563, PM: PM:24332216;PMC4040309.

[16] J.T. McBride, "The association of acetaminophen and asthma prevalence and severity," *Pediatrics* 2011;128:1181–1185.

[17] Joanne E. Sordillo, ScD*; Christina V. Scirica, MD, MPH; Sheryl L. Rifas-Shiman, MPH; Matthew W. Gillman, MD, SM; Supinda Bunyavanich, MD, MPH; Carlos A. Camargo Jr., MD, Phd; Scott T. Weiss, MD, MS; Diane R. Gold, MD, MPH; Augusto A. Litonjua, MD, "Prenatal and infant exposure to acetaminophen and ibuprofen and the risk for wheeze and asthma in children," *MPH Journal of Allergy and Clinical Immunology* February 2015, 135(2): 441–448.

conditions, but the ones who were later diagnosed with asthma were from families where other children had asthma, too. Asthma did not appear spontaneously in those who lacked the family tendencies.[18]

Likewise, Dutch researchers looked at an apparent association between children's asthma and a history of being taken into bed with their parents. They

> found no association between bed-sharing in early infancy and wheezing or diagnosis of asthma. By contrast, [they] found a positive association between bed-sharing in toddlerhood and both wheezing and asthma.[19]

Having taken three young kids into bed at various times, only one of whom ever developed asthma, I look at these figures and think that children wake up for different reasons at different ages, and parents comfort them out of a combination of sympathy and self-defense. That said, wakefulness among older children can be a symptom of undiagnosed asthma. So with toddlers, sharing a bed is not necessarily the cause of asthma, but it could be an indicator that asthma is already present.

When I read studies like the above, and all the corollaries of allergic disease with hygiene and affluence, I sometimes think we have been jumping back and forth over the same fence forever. Mark Jackson writes of an 18th century British physician named Thomas Withers who ascribed asthma and other conditions to something very like the current epidemic of progress.

> The greater irritability and weakness of the constitution in these days, may, in some measure, account for the greater frequency of the Asthma, especially if we add the inventive genius, and the rapid progress of mankind in all the various arts of modern luxury and refinement.

[18] A.K. Ortqvist, C. Lundholm, H. Kieler, J.F. Ludvigsson, T. Fall, W. Ye, C. Almqvist, "Antibiotics in fetal and early life and subsequent childhood asthma: Nationwide population based study with sibling analysis," *BMJ* 2014; 349: g6979, DOI: 10.1136/bmj.g6979.

[19] M.P. Luijk, A.M. Sonnenschein-van der Voort, V.R. Mileva-Seitz, P.W. Jansen, F.C. Verhulst, A. Hofman, W.W. Jaddoe, J.C. de Jongste, M.H. van IJzendoorn, L. Duijts, H. Tiemeier, "Is parent-child bed-sharing a risk for wheezing and asthma in early childhood?" *European Respiratory Journal* March 2015; 45(3): 661–669, DOI: 10.1183/09031936.00041714.

Jackson sums it up, "Along with gout and other nervous conditions, asthma had been effectively reformulated by Enlightenment physicians as one of the cardinal diseases of civilization." European history is a ping pong match of causation theories and treatments, including a period in France when Chinese culture was in vogue and various herbal teas entered the asthma formulary.

The modern epidemic of asthma is driven in part by different allergens in different parts of the world. Dr. Thomas Platts-Mills traces the exponential rise in child asthma in the United States to the year 1955 when children started sitting indoors in the afternoons to watch a particular television show instead of playing outside, and dust mites became the prevailing allergen. Unlike ragweed, which was seasonal, dust mites were year round.[20] North of the Arctic Circle in Sweden, according to Matthew Perzanowski, PhD, the dominant allergen is pet dander. It is too cold and too dry for dust mites but people have lots of dogs and cats, and the houses are well sealed against the brutally cold air.[21] In temperate climates, asthma triggered by diesel fumes is rampant near highways and buildings that burn dirty oil for heat.

Just as there is no single answer to why everyone who shows asthma symptoms has them, there is no single treatment, and there certainly is no cure. A good allergist will manage the variations using not only steroids but a palette of medications such as the mast-cell stabilizer called cromolyn, anti-leukotriene medications like montelukast (better known as Singulair), and very expensive regular injections of an anti-IgE medication omalizumab (Xolair). Like corticosteroids, these medicines have their limitations, which may only be revealed as they are used by ever-larger numbers of patients. For example, montelukast has been cited for mood disorders including suicidal ideation in children. The Food and Drug Administration recommends that long-acting β-agonists should not be administered without inhaled steroids, and that they should not be used as a rescue medication during an asthma

---

[20] Thomas A.E. Platts-Mills, MD, PhD, FRS, "The allergy epidemics: 1870–2010," *Journal of Allergy and Clinical Immunology* July 2015; 136(1): 3–13.

[21] Hayley James, BS; Matthew S. Perzanowski, PhD; Eva Ronmark, PhD; Bo Lundback, MD, PhD; Jillian Roper; Thomas A.E. Platts-Mills, MD, PhD, FAAAAI, "IgE antibodies to cat and cat components in relation to asthma in a population study of 963 18-year-olds from six schools in Northern Sweden," *Journal of Allergy and Clinical Immunology* February 2014; 133(2), Supplement: AB100.

attack. Asthma treatment also requires personal discipline, such as avoiding triggers, diligent cleaning, and restricting outdoor activity when ozone levels or pollen counts are high.

For all that asthma has been recognized and studied for hundreds of years, it is still not easy to diagnose. The best method — methacholine challenge — involves inhaling a chemical in escalating doses over two hours, which prompts the bronchia in the lungs to constrict, and measuring the effects on exhaled breath. Another method is to take samples of lung sputum and count the eosinophils, which indicate a level of allergic activity. No eosinophils, no allergic, steroid-responsive asthma. But these tests are cumbersome as well as time consuming, and a particular burden for children. A newer and less invasive method is to measure the level of fractional exhaled nitric oxide (FeNO) in exhaled breath using a portable machine called a NioxMino. FeNO is a byproduct of asthmatic inflammation.

For all the phenotypes and all the sophistication of diagnostics, millions of patients are misdiagnosed, or prescribed certain medications in sweeping one-size-fits-all expediency by non-specialists and specialists alike. They are not taught to monitor their own asthmatic status by blowing into a peak flow meter, or they neglect to visit their doctor. Instead they rely on the inhaled short-acting β-agonist albuterol rescue medication when they wheeze or persist with high doses of steroids even when their asthma is under control. As of this writing, another dismal wrinkle has emerged from the asthma swamp — the tendency of overweight children to treat every episode of short breath with their medication, which exacerbates their ill health instead of getting at the cause.

Contrast this with the TCM view, which seems to have recognized much sooner a range of phenotypes. A text called *Chinese Acupuncture and Moxibustion*[22] describes two broad asthma types — "excess" and "deficiency."

> Wind-cold type [a subset of excess] denotes asthma due to invasion of wind cold, which impairs the smooth flow of the lung qi, injures the skin and hair, and makes the pores closed. Since the lung and the superficial

---

[22] Cheng Xinnong, editor, *Chinese Acupuncture and Moxibustion* 2010; Foreign Language Press, Beijing.

defensive system are weakened, the lung qi fails to disperse and descend, leading to cough.

Manifestations of this type are:

> Cough with thin sputum, rapid breathing, accompanied by chills, fever, headache, and anhidrosis (inability to sweat) at the early stage, absence of thirst, white tongue coating, superficial and tense pulse.

Another subset of excess is "phlegm-type heat" whose manifestations are

> Rapid and short breathing, strong and coarse voice, cough with thick yellow sputum, sensation of chest stuffiness, fever, restlessness, dryness of the mouth, thick yellow or sticky coating, rolling and rapid pulse.

The trapping of "phlegm fire" gathering in the lungs, which sounds like bronchoconstriction, results in "chest stuffiness...fever, restlessness and dryness of the mouth... ." There are also herbal treatments, which will be discussed later in conjunction with Dr. Li's research.

Without digging too deeply into either approach, Western and Eastern, I am struck by the contrasts. In the former, the lungs are regarded as an organ detached from the upper airways, although usually not by allergists. We recognize the connection between allergic diseases of the skin, the airways, and the digestive tract as part of the so-called atopic or allergic march, but we do not treat them in concert, focusing variously on symptoms of one or the other. The Chinese approach is to not only correlate the symptomatic organs but to tie their malfunction to other organ systems that are apparently out of the picture.

The Yellow Emperor's Classic of Medicine illuminates symptoms and phenotypes that without too much imagination might be at home in the consulting room of a mainstream Western allergist. For example, "Huang Di" asks about patients who are fine when sitting or standing, but wheeze when lying down. "Others breathe coarsely upon exertion and still others have difficulty sleeping." A good case history by a modern allergist will extend to circadian rhythms, wakefulness as a symptom of poorly controlled asthma, and "exercise-induced asthma."

"Qi Bo" explains the role of the kidney thus:

> When the kidneys are diseased and the bladder cannot excrete, water stagnates. Then it moves back upward and distresses the lungs and bronchioles. When the patient lies down, the water blocks off the bronchioles, causing asthma.

Somehow, the poetry of Chinese medicine captures something that Western medicine does not.

In the book *Formulas and Strategies*, a book known to American students of TCM as "the Bensky" after one of its authors, you search futilely for the word "asthma", and instead find an alternative way of thinking about a range of symptoms.

While striking differences exist, the common denominator for converting the insights of one system into the benefits of the other is the underlying biochemistry. If herbal medicines can be made from things like *Zi Su Zi* and *Ting Li Zi*, it does not matter whether we use their Chinese names or their Greek names — *Perilla frutescens* and *Descurainia Sophia* respectively — everyone can be helped no matter what language they speak.

Changing Face of FDA Regulation

The integration of TCM with Western science is complicated not just by language, but by different worldviews that extend to the realm of how drugs are cleared for treatment. Regulators do not give up their standards of proof lightly, even if there is evidence of efficacy for a particular treatment.

Dr. Scott Sicherer said some things for my previous book that illuminate these differences in very commonsensical terms. First, that in China, what we call traditional Chinese medicine is just medicine. Second, the Western approach is to see the effects of one molecule on one other molecule, whereas in the Chinese medicines, multiple molecules interact with multiple other molecules. Our pharmaceutical companies look for drugs that work on a lone cytokine among the key asthma villains in the hope that after years of meticulous research they will make billions of dollars a year. But the question remains if targeting one cytokine at a time will be enough.

Chinese herbal medicines are at a disadvantage. How do you prove the medical efficacy of compounds for which there is strong promise without sacrificing the safeguards built into the existing medical system?

Standardization is important for generation of reproducible results and required for Food and Drug Administration (FDA) clinical studies. However, standardization of Chinese herbal formulas proves extremely challenging because the mixtures of herbs contain many constituents that are not clearly defined and they often contain many herbs.

Standardization of Herbal Product

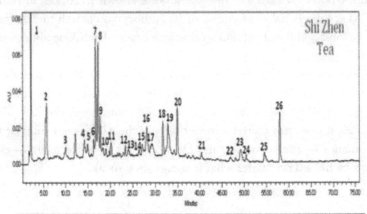

HPLC fingerprint of the internal herbal medicine.

After years of discussion, in 2000, the FDA recognized the importance of the movement toward alternative medicine by issuing the Guidance for Industry Botanical Drug Products, which states that active constituents in a botanical drug might not need to be identified when studying an investigational new drug if this is shown to be infeasible. Instead, the FDA will rely on other tests, including chromatographic fingerprints, chemical assays of characteristic markers, and biological assays, to ensure the quality, potency, and consistency.

In this changing regulatory landscape, Dr. Li and her colleagues began to explore the possibility of applying the lessons of thousands of years of Chinese medicine to a modern global epidemic.

The challenges were laid out. To be judged effective, an herbal medicine would have to equal or surpass the established treatments. At a minimum, a herbal therapy would have to do the thing that steroids do well. That is, suppress inflammation. But since steroids fall short or are even counterproductive in other areas, some of which have already been mentioned, there were the makings of a long-term agenda for experimentation for an herbal therapy.

These include:

Effects on constriction of the smooth muscles that line the airway, i.e., the airway smooth muscles (ASM). In standard asthma therapy, an additional medication called a beta-2 agonist is used in addition to steroids. These drugs are cited in black box warnings for such drugs as Advair and Symbicort.

Immunomodulation — steroids are known to have detrimental effects on the adrenal cortex, which results in suppression of immunity to infections as well as asthmatic inflammation. Patients get more colds and other infections and they are slower to recover from them. These tendencies can be measured by the appearance of certain cytokines.

Growth and weight gain — chronic systemic steroids suppress children's growth rates and cause patients to gain substantial amounts of weight.

Mood disorders — Patients with moderate to severe asthma suffer from both anxiety and depression, and steroid treatment appears to double the cytokines associated with these disorders.

Identification of active ingredients and their specific effects on the mechanisms of asthma.

Studying the synergistic effects of multi-herbal treatments compared to individual components.

Studying the effects on neutrophilic (non-allergic) inflammation which do not respond to steroids, as well as eosinophilic-dominated inflammation.

First Things First — A Murine Model for Asthma Research

First, they needed a surrogate for human subjects. Asthma occurs naturally in only two animals — cats and horses. One percent of cats, and an unknown number of horses — depending on how they are stabled and fed — develop a condition comparable to human asthma, but even if asthma were artificially induced in the laboratory, as it is with mice, neither species would be a suitable surrogate for study for public relations purposes if nothing else.[23]

In 1999, the Mount Sinai team joined by colleagues at Johns Hopkins, where Dr. Li and other Sinai doctors had worked till 1997, set out to induce asthma in mice, a well-established stand-in for the human immune system. They chose a strain of mice called AKR mice because of the availability of the conalbumin-specific Th2 clone (D10 G4.1), which allowed them to demonstrate the direct contribution of Th2 cells to allergic asthma in the mice themselves, not just in the test tube. The allergic airway and immune responses generated, including airway hyper-responsiveness, pulmonary eosinophilia, mucous hyperplasia, and increased Ag-specific IgE and Th2 cytokines, mimic those of human asthmatics, meaning any results in mice could hopefully be extrapolated to what occurs in humans.

Feasibility — Can a Herbal Treatment Work without Ephedra?

Earlier studies of *Xiao Qing Long Tang*, also known as Minor Bluegreen Dragon Concoction, did mitigate anaphylactic symptoms in animal studies, but it contains *Ma Huang*, whose Greek name *Ephedra Sinica* is a clue to its unsuitability. Ephedra makes this concoction unacceptable for human use in the United States because of many deaths linked to usage in diet treatments, including that of a professional baseball player, and also because it can be used to manufacture methamphetamine.

A 14-herb formula derived from *Ja Wai San Zi Tang* (now used at the China-Japan Friendship Hospital in Beijing) was chosen instead. For research it was registered as the investigational drug MSSM-002. All the herbs are prescribed as medicines in China and as employed in MSSM-002, are within ranges designated by the Pharmacopoeia of The People's Republic of China. The study would compare the efficacy of the drug and also compare it to the steroid dexamethasone (DEX), which is a standard asthma treatment.[24]

---

[23] Kevin Mullane, Michael Williams, "Animal models of asthma: Reprise or reboot?" *Biochemical Pharmacology* 2014; 87: 133.
[24] Xiu-Min Li, MD; Chih-Kang Huang, MS; Teng-Fei Zhang, PhD; Ariel A. Teper, MD; Kamal Srivastava, BS; Brian H. Schofield, JD; Hugh A. Sampson, MD, "The Chinese herbal

The mice were divided into four groups. Allergic asthma would be induced in three of them and one would be treated with the herbal medicine. The second would be treated with steroids. The third would be sham treated — i.e., sensitized but not receive any treatment. The fourth would be naïve — neither sensitized nor treated.

The mice were initially sensitized with two intraperitoneal (into the body cavity) injections containing conalbumin (CA), an egg protein antigen, and alum, a common adjuvant (one week apart). Seven days after the second injection, the mice were anesthetized and challenged intratracheally with more of the egg protein on days 20 and 30 after the process began.

Three days after the last intratracheal challenge with the conalbumin antigen came the time to assess whether the mice were indeed asthmatic. Rather than listen closely to hear their little lungs wheezing and coughing, airway responsiveness was tested after anesthesia and an intravenous injection of acetylcholine, followed by measuring the force of their exhaled breath. For people, this is done with an instrument called a peak flow meter.

After these figures were recorded, the mice were sacrificed and their blood analyzed to look for analogues for their respective state of airway hyper-responsiveness — that is, how impaired their breathing was because of their asthma — and the differences between the various categories of treatment and non-treatment. These measures were cells harvested from fluid squirted into and then collected (bronchoalveolar lavage fluid, or BALF), along with cells from the blood, and from the spleen. The cytokine interferon gamma IFN-γ and the antibody IgG2a were associated with less allergy, and therefore less asthma. The interleukins IL-4, IL-5, and IL-13 and the antibody IgE specific to the milk allergens were associated with more.

Three days after the last antigen challenge, AHR (airway hyper-reactivity) was measured as the airway pressure changes over time after acetylcholine challenge. The results are expressed as the airway pressure–time index (APTI), defined as the time-integrated change in peak airway pressure. The higher the values of APTI, the poorer the airway function. APTI levels of

medicine formula MSSM-002 suppresses allergic airway hyperreactivity and modulates TH1/TH2 responses in a murine model of allergic asthma," *Journal of Allergy and Clinical Immunology* 2000; 106(4): 660–668.

mice that were sensitized but sham treated were markedly higher than those of naïve mice. APTI levels in those that had been treated with both the herbal medicine and steroids were significantly lower and were essentially the same as those in naïve mice. These results demonstrated that, compared with sham treatment, the herbal preparation and steroids virtually eliminated AHR in this model. The herbal treatment was just as effective as the steroid treatment for airway function.

Some mice could breathe better than others, but that is not the sole measure of the effects of inflammation. Eosinophils, one of many kinds of white blood cells, are drawn to tissue that has experienced significant allergic activity. "Activated eosinophils are equipped with uniquely toxic molecules that they synthesize and store in intracellular granules, many of which can promote allergic inflammation…."

Eosinophils are a potent defense against helminths — parasites — and when they dump the contents of their toxic granules into surrounding tissues, they contribute to changes in the lung tissues, called airway remodeling. They are like landmines leftover after a battle. Elsewhere in the body, such as the esophagus, the effects of eosinophils releasing granules eventually cause a form of remodeling called fibrostenosis, which hardens and narrows the esophagus, making swallowing more difficult.

By counting the number of cells and the percentage of eosinophils in the bronchial fluid — BALF — the researchers determined that as with AHR, both steroid-treated and herbal-treated groups had statistically equivalent levels of these cells at levels roughly half that of the 44% of eosinophils in the sham-treated. Naïve mice showed virtually no eosinophils.

Mice from each group were necropsied — the lab equivalent of an autopsy. Major organs were presented to a pathologist who had no clue as to the experiment for observation of the state of the tissues. Except for the lungs, the pathologist saw no significant abnormalities. Again, the sham-treated, sensitized mice contained large numbers of eosinophils in the tissue surrounding the bronchia and blood vessels. There were also many mucus-secreting "goblet" cells and mucus plugs, particularly in the larger airways. By contrast, both herbal- and steroid-treated animals contained markedly fewer inflammatory cells, and while the number of goblet cells did not appear to be dramatically reduced by either treatment, neither showed airway mucus plugging.

Immediately after APTI measurement, the researchers determined the kinds of allergic (IgE) or allergy-blocking antibodies (IgG2a) that were produced, which is part of the immune system's humoral response. To do this, they pooled spleen cells isolated from four to six mice for each experimental group and cultured them (i.e., grew the cells in a dish) in complete culture medium, some in the presence of CA, the egg allergen. As expected, IgE levels were significantly, although not dramatically, decreased for mice treated with herbs, while IgG2a levels showed an increased trend toward significance from the sham-treated group. Steroid treatment also significantly decreased IgE levels but unlike the herbs, it also markedly reduced IgG2a levels. This is a key point, which, briefly, means that after steroid therapy, the lungs end up more allergic than before. (In addition, CA-specific IgG1 levels in both herb- and steroid-treated groups were also decreased compared with the sham-treated group.)

Beyond the humoral response, they looked at the cytokine profiles present in the different experimental groups — cytokines being the chemicals released by immune cells that broadly determine how the immune system will respond to a given stimulus, such as the allergen CA. A Th2 cytokine profile is associated with the allergic response. As expected, the herbal preparation down-regulated the production of Th2 cytokines, IL-4, IL-5, and IL-13, in cultured splenocytes. Because natural allergic airway reactions are likely mediated by a combination of Th2 cytokines, suppression of the three major Th2 cytokines by the herbal medicine may offer some advantage over the kind of single-antibody approach against IL-4, IL-5, IL-13 or their corresponding receptors, characteristic of so much laboratory research. Furthermore, the Th1 cytokine profile, necessary for fighting off various injections, was untouched.

As expected, Dex, the steroid, also suppressed antigen-induced AHR and eosinophilic inflammation in this model. However, in addition to suppressing Th2 responses (IL-4, IL-5, and IL-13/IgE), which is good, it suppressed Th1 responses (IFN-γ/IgG2a) — a negative collateral effect of suppressing the intended target, Th2. These findings suggest that MSSM-002, and perhaps other anti-asthma formulas, may offer relief from asthma without the well-known steroid side effect of leaving the patient infection prone.

The difference between the IgG2a levels is noteworthy because it points to a known weakness in steroid therapy — namely that it leaves the body more allergic. A healthy immune system has a vigorous Th1 profile, producing more IgG antibodies relative to Th2-induced, IgE antibodies. An allergic immune system is skewed toward a greater Th2/IgE antibody response over a Th1 response. As a side note, it is possible to have too much Th1 response, which results in autoimmune disease, but that is another discussion. The important point is that a healthy immune system will maintain an appropriate balance of Th1 and Th2 cytokines. Deviating too far in either direction leads to immune dysfunction. To develop tolerance to an allergen, you want to enhance the Th1 function over Th2 function in order to replace the IgE antibodies on effector cells with "blocking" antibodies — IgG2a in mice (IgG4 in people).

If steroids only suppress inflammation without encouraging the production of blocking antibodies, there is nothing to foreclose the possibility that allergenicity, and asthmatic inflammation, will rebound after treatment.

Dr. Engler's editorial reviewed the data and summarized its significance in a guest editorial published in the same issue of *The Journal of Allergy, Asthma and Clinical Immunology* (JACI). She not only analyzed the anti-asthma herbal medical intervention data approvingly, but signaled to her colleagues that Dr. Li's work represented a challenge to mainstream allergy practice, research, and to the laissez faire standards by which the supplement industry is regulated.

Citing the comparable effects to dexamethasone without the accompanying immune suppression, Dr. Engler writes,

> On the basis of the data, this complex herbal mixture cannot be dismissed as a mere placebo, a fact that is both exciting and threatening for allopathic practitioners and investigators. This courageous study represents a new frontier for clinical research in that the authors, working with an uncharacterized mixture in traditional pharmaceutical terms, tried to faithfully reproduce a mixture that has been clinically used in TCM practice.

She continues,

> Because by their nature herbal combinations cannot be easily standardized in terms of ingredients like currently licensed Food and Drug Administration–approved drugs can, developing a model and approach to testing complex and relatively crude "food supplement" materials that have

achieved public credibility is as important as the specific material in question.

The ubiquity of herbal supplements aimed at treating the immune system has created "popular perception… that these supplements are 'natural and safe'…. although increasing reports of adverse events have raised public awareness that natural is not risk free." She warns,

> For chronic asthma there are real concerns that the use of complementary or alternative medicine (CAM) may delay specific anti-inflammatory therapy and thereby increase risk of emergency visits and hospitalizations.

Dr. Engler adds that Dr. Li's article provides "a template for future testing of other … 'supplemental' asthma therapies." Finally,

> The article strengthens the need for a change in attitude within the medical profession to recognize the fact that medically efficacious therapies, from the patient's perspective, may come from arenas other than traditional allopathic medicine and pharmaceuticals.

In another study, the research team approached standardizing herbal formulas by using high-performance liquid chromatography (HPLC) fingerprinting and bioassay.[25]

All raw herbs used in the study were inspected for identity and quality by botanists trained in traditional Chinese herbology, in collaboration with Dr. Zhong Mei Zou at The Institute of Medicinal Plant Development, Chinese Academy of Medical Sciences, and Peking Union Medical College. Dr. Zou's institute used atomic absorption spectrometry and gas chromatography, respectively, to inspect each herb for possible heavy metal and pesticide concentrations according to quality and safety standards of the Pharmacopoeia of The People's Republic of China. Since MSSM-002 is prepared by extracting *Ling Zhi* (Ganodoma lucidum) separately from the

---

[25] Xiu-Min Li, MD; Teng-Fei Zhang, PhD; Hugh Sampson, MD; Zhong Mei Zou, PhD; Kirsten Beyer, MD; Ming-Chun Wen, MD; and Brian Schofield, JD, "The potential use of Chinese herbal medicines in treating allergic asthma," *Journal of Allergy, Asthma, and Clinical Immunology* August 2004; 93.

other 13 herbs and because the HPLC profile of *Ling Zhi* had previously been established, they focused on studying the 13 other herbs. Twenty-three diagnostic peaks were observed in their HPLC fingerprints. Two separate analyses found that the chromatographic fingerprints of MSSM-002 were reproducible.

The active constituents in the individual herbs or formulas that contribute to the inhibition of allergic airway responses had not yet been identified. Therefore, attention turned to characterizing complex formulations by a combination of chemical profiles and biological assays. Three separate experiments using 3 batches of MSSM-002 measured the effects on late-phase AHR as indicated by APTI measurements. Experiments 1 and 2 used freshly prepared liquid decoctions (traditional method). Experiment 3 used a lyophilized — freeze-dried — version, which would be an essential step for attempts to centrally manufacture, refine, and ship the medicines. Few of us would have the patience to boil our own fresh herbs. All three MSSM-002 preparations effectively and approximately equally reduced AHR after antigen challenge. An added finding — the lyophilized version could be stored for ten months with no loss of potency.

Simplifying Herbal Formulas

The question arises in many areas of engineering: how many moving parts does it take to get the job done? With herbal medicine, each additional ingredient adds to complexity of finding and processing herbs, monitoring their toxicity, and standardizing the formulation. Simplicity is an asset.

Although studies of food allergy herbal formula-2 (FAHF-2) found that a nine-herb formula (down from ten in the original *Wu Mei Wan* plus *Ling Zhi*, minus two alkaloids) was more effective than individual herbs, it remained an open question whether all 14 herbs in MSSM-002 were essential. The team hypothesized that some of the herbs in this formula might be superfluous.

Using the same murine model of allergic asthma to evaluate the actions of individual herbs on airway responses, they found that although no individual herbs were as effective as the whole formula, some, such as *Ku Shen*, were effective in suppressing AHR, whereas others, such as *Ling Zhi*, were effective in suppressing inflammation. Some, including *Gan Cao*, *Xin Ren*, and *Ge Gen*, had moderate effect on both AHR and inflammation, whereas others, such as *Dang Gui*, had little effect on AHR but a moderate effect on inflammation. One herb, *Da Zao*, actually increased AHR and eosinophilic inflammation.

Therefore, they formulated several simplified versions (MSSM-003, MSSM-003B, MSSM-003C, and MSSM-003D) based on the actions of individual herbs and theories of TCM formulation and compared them with the original formula. Further experiments showed that one combination, *Ling Zhi* (*Ganoderma lucidum*), *Ku Shen* (*Radix Sophora flavescentis*), and *Gan-Cao* (*Radix Glycyrrhiza uralensis*), suppressed AHR and eosinophilia as effectively as the original. It was dubbed ASHMI, for "anti-asthma herbal medical intervention." [26]

Multi-Year Research

In 2005, an application was submitted to the National Center for Complementary and Alternative Medicine (NCCAM), a division of the National Institutes of Health (NIH) for a Center of Excellence for Research on CAM (CERC) multi-year, multi-phase study to assess the safety and efficacy of ASHMI in people as well as determine how the herbs exert their function: PHS 398/2590 (Rev. 0501). The first two phases of this have now been completed and the third is ongoing.

This is a massive, highly deliberative process. Experiments are laid out in detail describing how many subjects, animal and human, will be involved, all the hypotheses and justifications for them, as well as all apparatus, methodologies, and statistical tools that will be used. The ideas must be novel, but not too novel, and the vision must be proven by accessible means. Each version of the proposal is read by experts, critiqued, and revised. A multi-year, multi-phase study like this one will be challenged along the way to justify release of funds.

The basic proposal describes a single, constant "administrative core" with the same people in charge of paperwork and compliance, as well as

---

[26] Paula J. Busse, MD; Brian Schofield, JD; Neil Birmingham, PhD; Nan Yang, PhD; Ming-Chuan Wen, MD; Teng Fei Zhang, PhD; Kamal Srivastava, MS; Xiu-Min Li, MD, "The traditional Chinese herbal formula ASHMI inhibits allergic lung inflammation in antigen-sensitized and antigen-challenged aged mice," *Annals of Allergy, Asthma and Immunology* March 2010; 104.

documenting results of all experiments and making the case for new ones that are suggested along the way.

The work consists of three principal projects, the first: to focus on investigating the pharmacological effects and immunotherapeutic mechanisms underlying the therapeutic effect of ASHMI using a murine asthma model; the second: to assess the effect of ASHMI treatment on atopic patients with moderate to severe persistent asthma; the third: to investigate how the three herbal components work together, and to explore the properties of each individual herb, to see how their constituents contribute to various biological effects.

During the time that this epic was being designed and fine-tuned, ASHMI was designated for study in collaboration between Dr. Li's Mount Sinai lab and Weifang Asthma Hospital, a chronic treatment center that draws patients from across China, where one of Dr. Li's former visiting scientists works. China, where all these herbs already had track records of safety and efficacy, as well as a serious epidemic of asthma, has a receptive regulatory climate for human studies of herbal medicines.

Patients were recruited from the outpatient facility in three steps: clinical history, clinical testing, and laboratory testing. Ninety-two atopic, non-smoking patients (43 men and 49 women, age 18–65 years) met the criteria of moderate-severe, persistent asthma and were admitted for the study. Inclusion criteria included a history of allergic asthma for at least one year; total serum IgE levels (above 100 IU/mL) indicating high Th2, allergic activity; daily asthma symptoms, exacerbations affecting activity and sleep; frequent symptoms at night, including poor lung function as well as poor lung function measured by force of exhaled breath; daily use of a beta-2-agonist (salbutamol/albuterol) in the past month; a history of reliance on systemic steroids. Briefly, these people were really ill with poorly controlled asthma.

Exclusion criteria included (1) use of oral corticosteroids, which dampen inflammation, within the previous four weeks (to ensure that they would have active inflammation at the start of the study); (2) heart, liver, kidney, or other organ diseases; (3) allergy or intolerance to the individual herbs in ASHMI; (4) pregnant and lactating women; and (5) being unable to comply with the research protocol because their asthma was so bad as to require acute treatment. The study was approved by the hospital medical ethics committee, and all patients gave written informed consent.[27]

Study Design

During the week prior to treatment, patients were allowed to use the b2-agonist and/or theophylline to avoid bronchoconstriction — they were not being treated for inflammation, but some of them needed help breathing. But any patient suffering exacerbations requiring additional medications would have been excluded from the experimental protocol. They were randomly assigned to receive ASHMI or prednisone with 46 subjects to each group. Subjects in the ASHMI group received oral ASHMI capsules (four capsules, three times a day) and placebo tablets similar in appearance to prednisone. Subjects in the prednisone group received oral prednisone tablets (20 mg once a day in the morning) and ASHMI placebo capsules for four weeks. For the duration of the study, leukotriene modifiers, antihistamines, and inhaled and intravenous glucocorticoids were prohibited, again with beta-2 agonist inhalation as needed.

Each ASHMI capsule contained 0.3 g dried aqueous extract. The total daily dose of 12 capsules (3.6 g) is equivalent to a raw-herb decoction of *Ling Zhi* (20 g), *Ku Shen* (9 g), and *Gan Cao* (3 g).

ASHMI capsules and ASHMI placebo capsules were prepared by Weifang Pharmaceutical Manufacturing Factory, affiliated with Weifang Asthma Hospital (major hospitals manufacture most of their own medications in China). Prednisone placebo tablets were made by Shandong Luoxin Ltd, Weifang. Before and after completing treatment, symptom scores, use of b2-agonist salbutamol, and lung function were evaluated. Total serum IgE, IL-5, IL-13, IFN-γ, and cortisol levels also were measured. Symptom scores, adverse events, and b2-agonist use were recorded daily. Grading of

---

[27] Ming-Chun Wen, MD; Chun-Hua Wei, MD; Zhao-Qiu Hu, MD, MS; Kamal Srivastava, MPhil; Jimmy Ko, MD; Su-Ting Xi, MD, MS; Dong-Zhen Mu, MD, MS; Ji-Bin Du, MD; Guo-Hua Li, MD; Sylvan Wallenstein, PhD; Hugh Sampson, MD; Meyer Kattan, MD; Xiu-Min Li, MD, "Efficacy and tolerability of antiasthma herbal medicine intervention in adult patients with moderate-severe allergic asthma," *Journal of Allergy and Clinical Immunology* September 2005.

adverse events followed the World Health Organization Recommendations for Grading of Acute and Subacute Toxicity. Hematology and serum chemistry testing and electrocardiograms were performed before and after treatment to measure any adverse effects.

Clinical and Laboratory Evaluation

Average daily symptom scores were evaluated over a one-week period before treatment to establish a baseline. Treatment was evaluated by analyzing average daily symptom scores in weeks 1, 2, 3, and 4 of treatment according to three categories: day time symptoms, night time symptoms, and allergic nasal and ocular symptoms and scored by physicians. Average daily use of short-term b2-agonists was evaluated over a one-week period before treatment and during the last week of treatment.

Forced expiratory volume (FEV1, the volume of air one can expel from one's lungs in the first second) and peak expiratory flow (PEF, the amount of air one can blow out when one tries to get rid of all of it) lung function measurements were recorded the day before treatment began and the day after it ended. All measurements were repeated three times, and the highest reading for each parameter was used for the study. Patients were not allowed to use theophylline 24 hours before or short-term b2-agonist six hours before lung function evaluation.

Venous blood samples were obtained from all patients before and after treatment to assess total serum IgE, peripheral eosinophil counts, cortisol levels, and serum IL-5, IL-13 and IFN-γ levels. To ensure consistency, all blood samples were drawn between 7:30 and 8:30 AM (before treatment and 48 hours after treatment).

Results

One patient in the ASHMI group dropped out of the study because of an unrelated infection in the fourth week of treatment. Forty-five patients in the ASHMI group and 46 patients in the prednisone group finished. There were no significant differences between the two groups in age, sex, asthma duration, or body weight before treatment. The baseline FEV1, PEF measurements, symptom scores, and use of b2-agonist in the two groups were no different. This ensured that these two groups were sufficiently similar so that any measured differences between them can be interpreted to be due to the treatment and not some extraneous factor.

Effects on Adrenal Function

Cortisol, our own natural anti-inflammatory hormone, is a useful marker for adrenal function. Cortisol production by the adrenal glands is at its highest point in the morning and lowest at night. This low level overnight is the reason that so many eczema patients suffer their worst itching after they go to bed. Their bodies are not protecting them from inflammation. Morning for adults and children normal ranges from 5–23 micrograms per deciliter (mcg/dL) and afternoon from 3–16 mcg/dL.[28]

People taking steroids long term to control inflammation experience a reduction in the adrenal glands' natural production of cortisol. In line with this, because everyone in the study had been taking steroids, cortisol levels were slightly below normal in both groups. After treatment, subjects in the prednisone treatment group showed a significant reduction in serum cortisol (5.1 + 3.0 to 3.7 + 2.3 mg/dL; P < .001). ASHMI patients on the other hand showed increased levels (5.4 + 2.8 to 7.7 + 2.3 mg/dL; P < .001), which were within the normal range.

Effects on Serum IgE and Serum Cytokine Levels

Total IgE levels were reduced by comparable amounts in both the ASHMI and prednisone groups (i.e., no significant statistical difference; p = .10). Serum IL-5 was significantly reduced in both, as were serum IL-13 levels; the prednisone group showed a more significant reduction than the ASHMI group, which could be advantageous. However, prednisone also reduced serum levels of the Th1 cytokine IFN-γ, while in the ASHMI treatment group, levels were significantly elevated after treatment. The difference between the groups was significant (P < 0.001). Higher levels of IFN-γ are associated with less allergy.

---

[28] http://www.webmd.com/a-to-z-guides/cortisol-14668?page=2

Safety

ASHMI and prednisone were well tolerated. Neither group showed abnormal findings in hematology, serum chemistry, or electrocardiograms, or exhibited serious adverse effects. Symptom scores showed similar improvement. Analysis of changes in symptom scores over weeks 1, 2, and 3 of treatment, however, revealed that improvement occurred earlier in the prednisone treatment group than in ASHMI group. Median symptom scores of ASHMI-treated patients were not significantly reduced until week 3 of treatment (baseline vs. weeks 1, 2, and 3 of treatment; median symptom scores were significantly reduced in patients treated with prednisone by week 1. A point to note is that the greater short-term potency of prednisone points toward the possibility of using ASHMI and prednisone together in cases where there is some urgency in treatment.

Effect on Pulmonary Function and B2-agonist Use

Breathing improved significantly after treatment, both with ASHMI and prednisone. Peak expiratory flow (PEF) values in both treatment groups also showed significant increases, although increases in FEV1 and PEF were significantly greater for the prednisone group than for ASHMI. Consistent with diminished symptoms and improved pulmonary function, inhaled b2-agonist use in both treatment groups declined, although the reduction was slightly greater in the prednisone-treated group.

Effect of ASHMI Treatment on Peripheral Eosinophils

Before treatment, eosinophil numbers in blood from both groups were slightly higher than the normal range. After treatment, peripheral eosinophils were significantly reduced with no significant differences between groups. By week 4 (last week of treatment) symptom scores for both were reduced by statistically equivalent levels.

Discussion

ASHMI registered substantial improvement in lung function measured in expiratory breath, but not as much as the prednisone-treated group.

Reduction in use of b2-agonist rescue medication, eosinophil counts, and serum IgE levels were comparable to prednisone. The study authors suggest these benefits are most likely because ASHMI works in people as it did in mice, completely blocking airway hyper-reactivity and markedly reducing eosinophilic inflammation in the lung. Direct effects on airway smooth muscle reactivity also may have been involved, because *ex vivo* studies (done on tissue outside the body) using murine tracheal rings with ASHMI showed inhibited airway smooth muscle contractility and enhanced muscle relaxation. Contraction of the tracheal rings is indicative of airway constriction.

Adverse effects were limited to a few instances of mild gastric discomfort. Prednisone patients showed significant weight gain after 4 weeks at levels roughly three times the ASHMI patients. Pretreatment serum cortisol levels were below normal in both groups. While the role of endogenous cortisol, i.e., produced by the body itself, in asthma is not settled, previous studies found that patients with asthma had lower cortisol levels than normal controls, possibly because of their asthmatic status and previous use of corticosteroids. In the study, as expected, serum cortisol levels were reduced by prednisone whereas, ASHMI treatment significantly increased serum cortisol levels to normal ranges after 4 weeks of treatment. These findings show that, although ASHMI and prednisone were almost equally effective in treating asthma symptoms, ASHMI had no negative effect on adrenal function.

Investigating the concomitant effects of ASHMI on nasal allergies — rhinitis — was not explicitly part of this study, although severity of allergic rhinitis was a factor in the total score as per the reference for symptom scoring.

High serum-total-IgE levels recorded before therapy were significantly reduced by both treatments. A previous study showed that *Gan Cao*, one ASHMI component, decreased IgE levels, but the effect of corticosteroids on IgE is still being debated. Another study found that subjects treated with 40 mg prednisone daily for a week, much less than at Weifang, had higher IgE levels. Another 33 found a transient increase in IgE levels after 15 days of oral prednisone, followed by a significant decrease after three weeks.

The balance of Th1 cytokines and Th2 cytokines for both atopy and asthma is considered crucial. Atopic individuals show a shift in immune responses away from a Th1 (IFN-γ) pattern toward Th2 (IL-4, IL-5, and IL-13) dominance. Numerous studies have shown that IL-4, IL-5, and IL-13 secretion after repeated antigen exposure is the major driving force behind persistent allergic asthma, suggesting that correcting the imbalance could be a cure. In this study, ASHMI treatment significantly reduced serum IL-13 and IL-5 levels while, unlike prednisone, increasing IFN-γ. These findings suggest that ASHMI, and perhaps other antiasthma herbal formulas, may offer some clinical advantages over corticosteroids.

Phase I Study

Building on the promising results at Weifang, the team initiated a phase I study to evaluate the hematologic tolerability and safety of ASHMI. A phase I (first-do-no-harm) study is the first step required by the US FDA for developing new botanical drugs. This was the first approval given by the agency for a botanical product to treat asthma.[29]

Despite strong public interest and increased use of complementary and alternative medicines (CAM), including TCM, there are few phase I studies of such treatments in the biomedical literature. The hurdles are many: standardization of the raw herbs, the manufacturing process, and the final product, as well as the safety data to ensure that pesticides, heavy metals, and microbes are below dangerous levels. All of which are key components in obtaining approval. This study employed a mandatory randomized double-blind, placebo-controlled, dose escalation design. The dose escalation approach ensures the safety and minimizes potential risks to study participants.

ASHMI was administered at three dosage levels to groups of four patients: 600 mg (two capsules); 1200 mg (four capsules); or 1800 mg (six capsules) twice a day for one week with two placebo subjects per group. Doses for the active group were increased after a review of safety data from subjects receiving the lower increment. If at any point a subject needed to be replaced and blinding was maintained, an additional subject would be recruited. If blinding could not be maintained, two additional subjects (one ASHMI and one placebo) were to be enrolled.

---

[29] Kristin Kelly-Pieper, MD; Sangita P. Patil, PhD; Paula Busse, MD; Nan Yang, PhD; Hugh Sampson, MD; Xiu-Min Li, MD; Juan P. Wisnivesky, MD, MPH; Meyer Kattan, MD, "Safety and tolerability of an antiasthma herbal formula (ASHMI™) in adult subjects with asthma: A randomized, double-blinded, placebo-controlled, dose-escalation phase I study," *Journal of Alternative and Complementary Medicine* 2009; 15(7): 735–743.

A total of 35 subjects with asthma underwent an initial screening evaluation and 14 subjects were excluded. Twenty subjects (12 on ASHMI and eight on placebo) completed the study and were included in the analysis. Although the protocol specified enrollment of 18 subjects in the study (six per dose level), because of an error in randomizing, two additional subjects were recruited in order to complete the middle dose cohort while maintaining blinding.

Subjects were started on ASHMI or placebo twice daily with meals for seven days. They continued their conventional asthma medications throughout the study, but were asked to refrain from other herbal medications. A daily diary was kept for morning and evening medication doses and peak flows, as well as any new symptoms. Investigators spoke by telephone to each subject twice during the study to reinforce medication compliance and assess reactions. During the final visit, the overall medical history was reviewed and physical examination, PEF, spirometry, electrocardiogram, and laboratory testing were repeated. Medication compliance was 98% in the ASHMI group and 96% in the placebo group.

No grade 3 adverse events occurred in subjects treated with ASHMI. (Grade 3 is defined as "severe" but short of "life-threatening", which is grade 4, grade 5 is death.) Three subjects receiving placebo had grade 3s. One had an elevated serum glutamic pyruvic transaminase and two subjects had electrocardiogram changes, although these were not considered clinically significant. Laboratory values after completing ASHMI treatment were within acceptable range compared to baseline. Three subjects had a minor decrease in bicarbonate levels (two treated with ASHMI and one in the placebo group).

Four subjects (33%) treated with ASHMI and four placebo-treated subjects (50%) reported gastro-intestinal symptoms. One placebo patient reported grade 2 transient vomiting, but most were grade 2 (mild to moderate, not requiring treatment). There were no acute asthma exacerbations.

Immunological Outcomes

Several measures of immune response and function were assessed, including select cytokine, chemokine, and growth factor production. All levels remained normal after one week of ASHMI. Pro-inflammatory cytokines such as tumor necrosis factor-alpha (TNF-a), interleukin (IL)-1, and IL-6 showed no increase, suggesting no harmful short-term immunologic impact.

The stage was set. With no harm indicated in the initial phase I study, further studies are underway to identify the active compounds in ASHMI, to further enhance quality control, and to perform a phase II study in humans, which will include evaluation of the drug's pharmacokinetics, i.e., how the body processes the drug after taking a dose.

While ASHMI showed promising results in both mice and men, three years after the Weifang study, its pharmacological and immunological actions had not been fully elucidated. In other words, it worked, but it is still unclear how it works. In 2008, researchers at Mount Sinai and Weifang and a pathologist prepared to test it on early- and late-phase airway reactivity [EAR and LAR] in mice, and investigate the underlying pharmacological and immunological mechanisms.

Mice were purchased and sensitized in the accustomed manner, with the appropriate control groups, then challenged and studied. The results were as follows:

ASHMI treatment abolished early airway reactivity and reduced histamine, LTC4 [leukotriene C4, a mediator associated with smooth-muscle contraction, pertinent to bronchoconstriction], and allergen-specific IgE levels. Airway reactivity was measured using peak expiratory flow [PEF], and measurements were performed 30 minutes after the 4th ovalbumin challenge. PEF of sham-treated mice was less than 50% of naïve mice, indicating severe bronchoconstriction while the ASHMI-treated group remained normal and slightly higher than naïve mice, demonstrating that ASHMI completely blocked early reactivity to allergen exposure. ASHMI-treated mice had significantly lower plasma and BALF histamine than sham-treated mice. ASHMI also significantly suppressed allergen-specific IgE synthesis whereas IgG1 and IgG2a levels were unaffected.

ASHMI did just as well with late airway reactions, and reduced airway inflammation and remodeling. APTI — respiratory distress following a challenge with acetylcholine — was measured two days after the 5th challenge. Sham-treated mice were significantly higher than naïve mice. However, APTI levels of ASHMI-treated mice were essentially the same as naïve mice. The percentage of eosinophils in BALF from the ASHMI-treated groups was significantly lower than in sham-treated mice. The fluid was also assayed for collagen production, associated with the process of airway remodeling, the long-term thickening of the smooth muscles of the bronchi. ASHMI-treated mice showed significantly less collagen production than sham-treated mice and were similar to naïve mice. Histological analysis showed that airways in sham-treated mice contained many goblet (mucus producing) cells, but not in the ASHMI-treated group. Infiltration of inflammatory cells was also reduced in ASHMI-treated mice.

BALF from sham-treated mice contained substantial levels of the allergy-related Th2 cytokines including IL-4, IL-5 and IL-13, which play a central role in orchestrating and prolonging airway inflammation. There was no corresponding effect on Th1 cytokine (IFN-γ), or T regulatory cytokines (IL-10 or TGF-β). The picture with ASHMI treatment was starkly different. IL-4, IL-5, and IL-13 were undetectable in BALF from ASHMI treated mice whereas IFN-γ, IL-10 and TGF-β were markedly elevated, indicating specific Th2 suppression and reduction of allergenicity.

By these and many other indicators, ASHMI was showing great promise in the laboratory. It effectively blocked the longer-term effects of asthma as indicated by several different measures.

How long will treatment last and what are the mechanisms critical to its success?

A newer study sought to test the persistence of ASHMI-mediated protection from allergic asthma and assess the functional contribution of two cytokines, IFN-γ and TGF-b, both of which were elevated after treatment, in affording this protection.[30]

The authors pointed out that the protective role of IFN-γ for allergies is well-known. Mice with deficient IFN-γ production show elevated AHR and specific IgE. In humans, low IFN-γ levels in early life were found to be a predictor of asthma.

ASHMI treatment commenced after the third ovalbumin (OVA) egg protein allergen challenge. Immediately after completing treatment, sham-treated mice showed sustained airway hyper-responsiveness upon re-challenge, with significantly higher APTI levels than naïve mice. By contrast,

---

[30] Tengfei Zhang, Kamal Srivastava, Ming-Chun Wen, Nan Yang, Jing Cao, Paula Busse, Neil Birmingham, Joseph Goldfarb, Xiu-Min Li, "Pharmacology and immunological actions of a herbal medicine ASHMI™ on allergic asthma," *Phytotherapy Research* 2010; 24: 1047–1055.

OVA/ASHMI mice had normal APTI levels. Resolution of airway hyper-responsiveness was total and furthermore, it did not return after re-challenges up to eight weeks after treatment stopped. Significantly, eosino-phil numbers remained persistently low eight weeks post-therapy, 48 hours after the final antigen challenge. Peribronchial inflammation, eosinophil count, and goblet cells in the airways were also reduced after eight weeks.

IFN-γ and TGF-b: Which is the Key Measure?

To study the effects of IFN-γ and TGF-b, ASHMI was administered to a new set of ovalbumin-sensitized mice for six weeks. The added layer of complexity to this experiment was to include antibodies that could block the function of IFN-γ or TGF-b in the mouse's body — dubbed anti-IFN-γ or anti-TGF-b. By blocking either of these molecules in the body, they could assess the specific function of naturally occurring IFN-γ and TGF-b. Anti-IFN-γ (clone H22, 100 mg/week, i.p.), anti-TGF-b (clone ID11, 100 mg/week, i.p.) antibodies, and appropriate isotype control antibodies were administered intraperitoneally to ASHMI or sham-treated mice, one day before treatment and then weekly for six weeks. All subjects (except naïve mice) were re-challenged as above up to eight weeks post-therapy. Forty-eight hours after the final OVA challenge, airway responses and cytokines were measured.[31]

Under an antibody neutralization protocol, ASHMI-treated mice and a sham-sensitized control group were given anti-IFN-γ antibodies, anti-TGF-b antibodies, or isotope-control neutral antibodies. Eight weeks post-therapy, mice treated with ASHMI supplemented by the anti-IFN-γ antibodies lost their protection from airway hyper-responsiveness, while those given the neutral antibodies did not. Anti-TGF-b or isotype control antibodies suf-fered no increase in airway hyper-responsiveness. Administration of anti-IFN-γ or anti-TGF-b Abs during treatment had no effect on APTI of naïve mice. Similarly, co-administration of anti-IFN-γ but not isotype control antibodies resulted in the loss of eosinophil suppression, whereas those that

---

[31] K. Srivastava, T. Zhang, N. Yang, H. Sampson, X.M. Li, "Anti-asthma simplified herbal medicine intervention-induced long-lasting tolerance to allergen exposure in an asthma model is interferon-γ, but not transforming growth factor-β dependent clinical and experimental allergy," *Clinical and Experimental Allergy* 2010; 40(11): 1678–1688.

received anti-TGF-b or isotype control antibodies maintained this protection. What this means is that IFN-γ, not TGF-b, is a crucial mediator of ASHMI's therapeutic response.

In the same issue of *Clinical and Experimental Allergy*, Yui-Hsi Wang, PhD, and Simon. P. Hogan PhD, of Cincinnati Children's Hospital Medical Center appraised Dr. Li's previous work favorably in an editorial with the whimsical and upbeat title, "Chinese anti-asthma tea to go!" They wrote,

> in a randomized, double-blinded, placebo-controlled, dose-escalation phase I study on allergic asthmatic patients and a randomized study in adult patients with moderate–severe allergic asthma, patients demonstrated good efficacy and tolerability of ASHMI™ and post-treatment lung function analyses demonstrated improved FEV1 and peak expiratory flow. Notably, the improvement in lung function was slightly but significantly greater than that of the conventional anti-asthma therapeutic prednisone. [32]

The commentators pointed out, however, that the earlier studies had not shed light on the underlying mechanisms, but that the new experiment did.

> Treatment of mice with ASHMI™ via drinking water for four weeks prevented the development of the experimental asthmatic symptoms. Notably, the reduction in the experimental asthmatic response in ASHMI™-treated mice was associated with the reduced levels of Th2 cytokines in the bronchoalveolar lavage fluid (BALF). Importantly, the authors demonstrated that the therapeutic effects exerted by ASHMI™ remained at eight weeks post-therapy.

They were encouraged enough by what results meant for allergic asthma to call for more study with non-allergic asthma.

Licorice to the Rescue?

Many recreational foods have medical origins. Anyone who likes a good martini can taste juniper and other botanicals, betraying gin's origins as a treatment for stomach aches among other ailments. It brings to mind the

---

[32] Y-H Wang and S.P. Hogan, "Chinese herbal anti-asthma tea to go!" *Clinical and Experimental Allergy* October 2010; DOI: 10.1111/j.1365-2222.2010.03621.x 1590–1592.

pronouncement by Homer Simpson: "Alcohol, the cause of and solution for all of life's problems."

I once chewed a pill of FAHF-2 — Dr. Li's food allergy herbal formula and found it quite bitter, but the aftertaste reminded me of that staple of Chinese cooking, five-spice powder. Licorice, *Glycyrrhiza uralensis*, is widely used in TCM for its properties of relieving cough and reducing asthma symptoms, and is one of the three herbs in ASHMI. But how does this substance, which is usually administered in sweet and sticky form under brand names including Twizzlers and Good and Plenty, deliver its healing properties?

Teasing out the contribution of these components was another collaboration between Mount Sinai and Weifang Asthma Hospital. The major chemical constituents in *Glycyrrhiza uralensis* are triterpenoids and flavonoids with anti-inflammatory effects. Dr. Li's team had previously isolated five flavonoids from *Glycyrrhiza uralensis* and compared the effects of these compounds to those of glycyrrhizin on secretion of eotaxin-1 by human fetal lung fibroblasts (HFL-1), which are better than adult lung fibroplasts for demonstrating gene expression, particularly the crucial regulatory cytokine, TGF-b.[33,34]

The flavonoids liquiritigenin, isoliquiritigenin and 7, 40-dihydroxyflavone (7, 40-DHF) suppressed eotaxin secretion more effectively than glycyrrhizin alone. Flavonoids, commonly found in foods, fruits, vegetables and beverages, are largely safe for human use, although licorice in large quantities does have side effects such as high blood pressure, low potassium levels, weakness, paralysis, and occasionally brain damage. The suppression of eotaxin secretion was particularly intriguing because this chemokine helps attract eosinophils. Hypothetically, decreasing eotaxin levels should reduce the primary offending culprit — eosinophils — in many cases of allergic asthma.[35]

---

[33] http://www.cellapplications.com/product-type/human-lung-fibroblasts-hlf?id=72

[34] Nan Yang, Sangita Patil, Jian Zhuge, Ming-Chun Wen, Jayaprakasam Bolleddula, Srinivasulu Doddaga, Joseph Goldfarb, Hugh A. Sampson, Xiu-Min Li, "*Glycyrrhiza uralensis* flavonoids present in anti-asthma formula, ASHMI™, inhibit memory Th2 responses in vitro and in vivo," *Phytotherapy Research* November 2012; 27: 1381–1391.

[35] http://www.webmd.com/vitamins-supplements/ingredientmono-881-LICORICE.aspx?activeIngredientId=881&activeIngredientName=LICORICE

When eosinophils are recruited for allergy duty, they leave the affected tissue scarred and rigid. The team hypothesized that if they could successfully suppress eotaxin secretion, these flavonoids might have anti-Th2 inflammatory effects. They set out to test the effects of liquiritigenin, isoliquiritigenin and 7, 40-DHF on effector memory Th2 cells (D10.G.4.1), a classical Th2 clone and also in a mouse model of allergic asthma.

In patients with chronic allergic asthma, effector memory Th2 cells produce abundant Th2 cytokines after encountering allergens, and they play a critical role in orchestrating and perpetuating inflammation in airways starting early in life. In mice with chronic asthma, these Th2 memory responses have been shown to last for over a year — half their life expectancy. This longevity is significant because it indicates that lungs can remain highly reactive even in the absence of exposure to their allergens. Patients get careless about using their controller medications — mainly steroids — when they are unsymptomatic.

D10 cells are "classical" effector memory Th2 cells. Previous research showed that ASHMI significantly inhibited IL-4 production by memory Th2 cells in a non-cytotoxic manner.[36]

The latest study investigated how three flavonoids previously isolated from *Glycyrrhiza uralensis* on memory Th2 effector cells could inhibit the secretion of the pertinent cytokines. The *in vitro* study — cells treated in a dish — showed that isoliquiritigenin, 7,40-DHF and liquiritigenin significantly suppressed production of IL-4 and IL-5, by antigen-stimulated D10 cells. 7, 40-DHF had the highest potency, and it accomplished this, moreover, without reducing cell viability of D10 cells even at the highest concentration used. This is a key point of difference between ASHMI and steroid-based treatments. Specifically, it reduces inflammation without compromising the overall immune system. Th2-driven immunity does have a role in health and we do not want it wiped out altogether, just reduced to its normal level of activity.

---

[36] Kamal Srivastava, MPhil; Ariel A. Teper, MD; Teng-Fei Zhang, PhD; Side Li, MD; Martin J. Walsh, PhD; Chih-Kang Huang, MS; Meyer Kattan, MD; Brian H. Schofield, JD; Hugh A. Sampson, MD; Xiu-Min Li, MD, "Immunomodulatory effect of the antiasthma Chinese herbal formula MSSM-002 J onTh2 cells," *Journal of Allergy and Clinical Immunology* 2004; 113(2).

After antigen stimulation 7, 40-DHF also inhibited D10 cell proliferation, reducing levels of the transcription factor GATA-3, which as previously stated does duty as the "commander" of Th2 function. When it becomes too powerful, it stops being merely part of a defense against powerful invading parasites and starts directing attacks on otherwise innocuous pollens and food proteins.

Consistent with the *in vitro* findings, even more important is that 7, 40-DHF treatment of OVA-challenged mice significantly inhibited IL-4 and IL-13 production by lung cells, which are instrumental in allergic and eosinophilic inflammation. Th2-derived cytokines are also key factors in directing IgE synthesis. Serum levels of these allergic antibodies were also significantly decreased. Unsurprisingly, however, treatment with a single component of ASHMI, even at double the amount present in the whole herb extract, does not replicate the effect of ASHMI. Combinations of herbs are essential to induce positive effects of ASHMI. Extracts of the two other herbs in ASHMI, *Radix sophorae flavescentis* and *Ganoderma lucidum* also inhibit Th2 cytokine production *in vivo*. The inhibited contraction of murine tracheal rings and increased production of the potent smooth muscle relaxant PGI2 by human bronchial smooth muscle cells appears to reside in *Radix sophorae flavescentis*, thus contributing to the reduction in AHR. ASHMI plays as a trio, not a collection of soloists.

The relative contributions of the three ASHMI components were further explored in "Constituents of the anti-asthma herbal formula ASHMI™ synergistically inhibit IL-4 and IL-5 secretion by murine Th2 memory cells, and eotaxin by human lung fibroblasts in vitro."[37]

Inhibiting secretions of these agents is particularly interesting because they are to eosinophils what chum is to shark fishing, attracting these potent cells to inflamed mucosal tissue. Bellanti *et al.* write that "[e]osinophils preferentially home to these tissues" because activation molecules are "upregulated by IL-4, IL-5, chemokines, e.g., eotaxins, and leukotrienes…"

They continue, "IL-5 is by far the most important eosinophil-specific factor as it is responsible for both eosinophil growth and differentiation

[37] Bolleddula Jayaprakasam, Nan Yang, Ming-Chun Wen, Rong Wang, Joseph Goldfarb, Hugh Sampson, Xiu-Min Li, "Constituents of the anti-asthma herbal formula ASHMI™ synergistically inhibit IL-4 and IL-5 secretion by murine Th2 memory cells, and eotaxin by human lung fibroblasts *in vitro*," *Journal of Integrative Medicine* May 2013; 13(3).

and release of eosinophils from the bone marrow." In military terms —
I know some people do not like them but when discussing the immune
system it is hugely convenient — IL-5's role in eosinophilic infiltration is
roughly like a general choosing new cadets at West Point and guiding their
careers all the way through training and assignment to a theater of combat
(Bellanti, p. 695).

In "Constituents…," the individual herb extracts were fingerprinted,
along with standard ASHMI, and an experimental form of the drug created
by recombining the individual extracts. Fifty mg of ASHMI (equivalent to
437 mg of raw herbs) was dissolved in water, and then extracted with
butanol five times. The combined extracts were dried and re-dissolved in 2
mL of 50% methanol. A total of 10 mL of the resulting solution was
injected into the HPLC system.

HPLC fingerprints showed that the combination of individual extracts
(experimental ASHMI) had a pattern consistent with the standard ASHMI,
which means that some lesser and simpler combination of the herbs may
prove as effective as the larger formula and be easier to produce at scale
without sacrificing effectiveness. The various formulations were employed in
a series of experiments.

ASHMI constituents exhibited synergy in suppressing memory Th2
cell IL-4 production D10 cells cultured with ASHMI and individual herb
extracts of *Ling Zhi, Ku Shen* and *Gan Cao* at different concentrations
inhibited production of IL-4, a key Th2 cytokine involved in allergic airway inflammation at levels consistent with concentrations. The highest
concentration tested (500 mg/mL) of ASHMI produced 75% inhibition.
The individual extracts also produced concentration-dependent inhibition
of IL-4 production. Synergy was even more pronounced at the lower
concentrations.

ASHMI constituents exhibited synergy in suppressing IL-5 production
by Th2 cells ASHMI constituents also exhibit synergy in suppressing production of IL-5, key to eosinophil activation. ASHMI and each individual
extract produced concentration-dependent inhibition of IL-5 production by
D10 cells.

ASHMI constituents exhibited synergy in suppressing eotaxin-1 production by HFL-1 cells. Eotaxin, together with Th2 cytokines, plays
an important role in mediating airway eosinophilic inflammation by

recruiting eosinophils to inflamed tissue. Lung fibroblasts are a major cellular source of eotaxin. HFL-1 cell has been widely used to investigate inhibition of eotaxin production. ASHMI and its constituents, *Ling Zhi*, *Ku Shen*, and *Gan Cao* showed concentration-dependent inhibition of eotaxin-1 production. ASHMI inhibited eotaxin-1 production almost completely at the highest concentration tested (500 mg/mL), as did *Ling Zhi* by itself.

Cell Viability

No cytotoxicity was detected in ASHMI or any individual herb-containing D10 cell culture at any concentration. ASHMI, *Ku Shen* and *Gan Cao* produced no toxicity in HFL-1 cultures. *Ling Zhi* reduced HFL-1 cell viability by 20% at the highest concentration tested (500 mg/mL).

When Standard Medication is Not Enough

Despite the general effectiveness of the combination of inhaled steroids and beta agonists, sometimes it does not work, as with steroid-resistant asthma. Another subset of asthmatic patients responds poorly to beta-2 agonists for a variety of reasons, such as differences in disease phenotype, body weight, and perhaps pharmacogenomic variations — genetic variations that affect an individual's response to drugs. Some develop tolerance to beta agonists after regular use. As mentioned, the long-term safety of beta-2 agonists has been controversial.

A new set of experiments set out to explore whether ASHMI could avoid some of the problems associated with beta agonists. Two sets of mice were sensitized with ovalbumin, as previously described, and one group was left naïve. Two hours before intravenous acetylcholine challenge, one group was "vehicle-treated," i.e., dosed with medication minus the active ingredient, and the other received a single dose of oral ASHMI. They were anesthetized, intubated and placed on special mouse respirators (which cost about $5,000 in case you're thinking about doing this at home) and their muscles paralyzed by IV injection. Airway pressure changes were recorded for four minutes. Airway hyper-responsiveness expressed as APTI values was significantly greater in vehicle-treated mice compared with naïve animals, indicating successful establishment of AHR. In contrast, APTI values of ASHMI-treated mice were dramatically lower than those of the vehicle group and essentially the same as those of naïve mice, meaning that ASHMI worked.[38]

A single acute oral dose of ASHMI dramatically reduced AHR in response to the acetylcholine challenge. The size of the response was dose dependent. Examination of the tissues — *ex vivo* experiments — showed that the reaction ASHMI significantly increased was secretion of tracheal ring prostaglandin E2 (PGE2), also called dinoprostone. PGE2 suppresses T cell receptor signaling and may contribute to the resolution of inflammation.

The primary findings of the study were that ASHMI inhibits airway constriction when given orally to OVA-sensitized mice or by *ex vivo* exposure of tracheal rings from the same mice. These effects were dose dependent, and, in *ex vivo* experiments, reversible after wash-out. Citing other findings that involved inhaled PGE2 reducing allergen-induced bronchoconstriction, methacholine responsiveness, and aspirin-induced bronchoconstriction asthmatics, the authors say there is renewed interest in targeting EP4 receptors for bronchodilator therapy.

Thus ASHMI treatment may help improve on the current generation of bronchodilators.

> Our study results suggest that ASHMI may be a valuable oral asthma drug that could potentially provide relief from bronchoconstriction, especially in patients responding poorly to beta agonists due to genetic reasons or those who have become tolerant after chronic use.

Neutrophil-Dominant Asthma

Corticosteroids are the medication of choice for eosinophil-dominant asthma, but in most severe cases, another inflammatory cell, the neutrophil, is dominant. These are the most abundant white blood cells, and steroids are

---

[38] Kamal Srivastava, Hugh A. Sampson, Charles W. Emala, Sr, Xiu-Min Li, "The anti-asthma herbal medicine ASHMI acutely inhibits airway smooth muscle contraction via prostaglandin E2 activation of EP2/EP4 receptors," *American Journal of Physiology — Lung Cellular and Molecular Physiology* 2013; 305: L1002–L1010.

seen as essentially useless against them. Neutrophils are both early recruits to the airways in an allergen exposure and plentiful in the late phases as well.

As an infection-fighting cell they surround microbes and viruses and secrete toxins. Another mechanism is the construction of neutrophil extracellular traps [NETs] out of their own DNA. These surround the infectious agent, creating a compartment in which the extermination can go on somewhat shielded from healthy adjacent tissue. Neutrophils are deemed to contribute to airway remodeling, perhaps because when they are drawn to inflammation, they are "sequestered, accumulated, and activated into the microvasculature."

There is something of a chicken-and-egg argument about the role of steroids in neutrophilic asthma. As the study's authors note:

> Because neutrophils are relatively steroid-resistant, it was hypothesized that this increased neutrophilic inflammation might explain the poor response to corticosteroids seen in severe refractory disease. It could be argued, however, that the increased presence of neutrophils in severe asthma may be the result of treatment with high-dose corticosteroids rather than a manifestation of the disease itself.

Whatever the specifics of how neutrophils work, and whether they thrive in the presence of corticosteroids or because of it, a substantial percentage of severe asthma evades conventional treatment. The Sinai team hypothesized that ASHMI and some of its active compounds might help. Further, they hypothesized that TNF-a, IL-8, and IL-17, all critical to underlying mechanisms of neutrophilic inflammation, might be regulated by ASHMI. If ASHMI could succeed with neutrophilic asthma, it would represent a real breakthrough.

They used a ragweed asthma model characterized by the presence of both eosinophils and neutrophils called "mixed granulocytic airway inflammation." While both cells are present, neutrophils predominate. Ragweed has several advantages over the ovalbumin-based models. It do not require prolonged aerosolized exposures every day, or use of an adjuvant for airway challenges. Elevated APTI values after acetylcholine challenge indicated that ragweed-sensitized mice had much worse airway sensitivity than the alum control (those that received only the adjuvant) and naïve mice. ASHMI-treated mice exhibited marked reductions in AHR when compared with those that were sensitized but sham-treated. This model, demonstrated that

ASHMI treatment significantly suppressed both neutrophil and eosinophil airway inflammation via regulation of associated chemokines and cytokines. In addition, AHR, mucous production, and ragweed-specific IgE all fell significantly, whereas steroid treatment reduced BAL fluid eosinophil percentage but failed to decrease neutrophil numbers or decrease AHR.

A Scientist's Work is Never Done

A further multi-year phase of this research is beginning, to encompass mouse studies and also a multi-ethnic set of human subjects. One of the most intriguing elements is interplay between the innate immune system and the acquired immune system that makes it so hard to distinguish infectious disease from allergic disease, resulting in much ineffectual or counterproductive treatment. When you get stung by a bee for the first time, you will have an uncomfortable reaction no matter who you are, but if you are prone to allergies, your body might start making antibodies that will make the next sting a lot worse. When I am walking down my Brooklyn street I have to ask myself, "Am I sneezing because the trees are getting ready to flower or because the bus that just went by was spewing black exhaust?" Parents and patients everywhere have to ask themselves, is that wheezing and coughing causes by allergies, by a virus, or because that the wind is blowing from that chemical plant in the next town? And then they have to wonder, how long will it take for the Fluticasone inhaler to kick in?

The eosinophilic phenotype likely reflects ongoing adaptive immunity in response to an allergen in which the Th2 cytokines IL-4, and IL-5 play a key role, IFN-γ (produced by Th1 cells) down regulates this response, which is also influenced by Tregs that secrete regulatory cytokines, including IL-10. The neutrophilic phenotype is thought to reflect innate immune system activation, i.e., our first line of defense, in response to pollutants or infectious agents.

ASHMI and Mental Health

That there should be a connection between asthma and mood disorders should surprise no one. Shortness of breath, poor blood oxygenation resulting in loss of mental sharpness and energy, feelings of suffocation, sleepless nights followed by sleepy days are all consequences of poorly controlled asthma. Adults with asthma (7.5%) suffer serious psychological distress at a rate more than double that of the overall US population (3.0%) and adults without asthma (2.6%).

The disease does not have to even be considered physically debilitating to affect mood. A study of adults at one Texas medical center showed that among the 9% diagnosed with asthma, most of it "predominantly mild" who rated their health as good or excellent, the risk of anxiety was 43.5%.[39]

Younger asthmatics also suffer. Twenty to 40% of asthmatic adolescents experience significant symptoms of anxiety.[40]

A 2015 study of 720 adolescents with current asthma (5.2% of the total sample), reported depression symptoms, cigarette smoking, and cocaine use occurred more frequently than those without asthma. Substance abuse increased with depression; among youth with asthma: 20% reported suicidal ideation, 40% had smoked cigarettes, 67% had smoked marijuana, 37% had engaged in binge drinking, and 12% had used cocaine in the past 30 days.[41]

The Young and Well Cooperative Research Centre in Australia, which has one of the highest asthma rates in the world, drew an explicit connection between asthma, depression, and anxiety for young people:

The mental health and well-being of the young people surveyed was poor. This was particularly the case for young people whose asthma was poorly controlled. Just over 50% of those who participated in the study had K10 (Kessler Psychological Distress Scale) scores, which suggest they are likely to have a mental disorder, this is double the rate in the wider population of young people. Participants cited a number of concerns that impacted

---

[39] Elan Gada, MD; David A. Khan, MD; Laura F. DeFina, MD; E. Sherwood Brown, MD, PhD, "The relationship between asthma and self-reported anxiety in a predominantly healthy adult population," *Annals of Allergy, Asthma and Immunology* April 2014; 112(4):329–332.

[40] Sangita P. Patil, Changda Liu, Joseph Alban, Nan Yang, Xiu-Min Li, "*Glycyrrhiza uralensis* flavonoids inhibit brain microglial cell TNF-α secretion, p-IκB expression, and increase brain-derived neurotropic factor (BDNF) secretion," *Journal of Traditional Chinese Medical Sciences* July 2014; 1(1): 28–37.

[41] Bruce G. Bender, PhD, "Depression symptoms and substance abuse in adolescents with asthma," *Annals of Allergy, Asthma and Immunology* October 2007; 99(4): 319–324. http://www.annallergy.org/article/S1081-1206(10)60547-9/fulltext

their health and well-being, including self-consciousness, lack of confidence and poor body image.[42]

To make matters worse, there is the strong correlation between asthma and obesity, attributed to such mechanical effects as "inflammation associated with airway narrowing, increased airway reactivity to environmental allergens, and, more recently, disruption of the autonomic nervous system mediated by leptin."[43] Whatever the mechanisms, obesity seldom improves anyone's state of mind. Regular use of steroids, particularly prednisone, also contributes to weight gain from fluid accumulation, among other things.

Part of the problem is surely psychological — being chronically ill can make you feel miserable. But part of it is also biochemical and concomitantly, the medicines most effective at controlling asthma are not equally effective at instilling joy in everyday living. For example, montelukast, the leukotriene agonist, which was once hailed as a wonder drug, especially for children because it could be taken orally, has been tied to mood swings including "suicidal ideation" in large enough numbers to have warranted study, although without any conclusive findings as to the mechanisms. Higher levels of anxiety in asthmatic patients correlate with high concentrations and long-term use of inhaled corticosteroids. The problems with systemic steroids are worse. My own experience in online groups of asthmatics that require regular use of prednisone has shown me very poor quality of *vivre* and no *joie*.

That the biochemistry of asthma affects mental health is unsurprising. Neuroscientist Jessica Martin, PhD, has written about the overlap of the nervous system with asthma: While asthma is recognized as an inflammatory condition stemming from a skewed immune system, many of the hallmark symptoms, such as bronchoconstriction (a decrease in size of the airway openings), are in fact mediated in part by the cells of the nervous system (i.e., neurons). The lungs contain nerve cell endings that can sense chemical irritants. If a chemical activates these neurons, the information is relayed and

---

[42] M. Blanchard, J. Morris, E. Birrell, J. Stephens-Reicher, A. Third, J. Burns, *National Young People and Asthma Survey: Issues and Opportunities in Supporting the Health and Wellbeing of Young People Living with Asthma* 2014; Young and Well CRC, Melbourne.

[43] Emilio Arteaga-Solis, MD, PhD; Meyer Kattan, MD, "Obesity in asthma: Location or hormonal consequences?" *Journal of Allergy and Clinical Immunology* May 2014; 133(5): 1315–1316.

integrated into the central nervous system, which can then send a signal back through a different set of neurons to the muscles lining the airways. The muscles are commanded by these neurons to contract and airways constrict. For a person with asthma, the same amount of a chemical irritant causes a much greater airway constriction than someone without asthma. Thus, an asthmatic's airways are said to be "hyperreactive" and wheezing ensues.[44]

In a study published in 2014, the Mount Sinai team explored the potential of several flavonoids in ASHMI for their effects on the biochemistry of mood. ASHMI had been shown to inhibit peripheral TNF-a secretion in asthmatic mice. High TNF-a levels not only stimulate mucus production and mucus gene expression in the peripheral system; in the central nervous system, elevated TNF-a is also associated with anxiety/depression, whereas an important nervous system neuropeptide, brain-derived neurotropic factor (BDNF) has anti-depressant effects. *Glycyrrhiza uralensis* flavonoids inhibit brain microglial cell TNF-a secretion, p-IkB expression, and increase brain-derived neurotropic factor (BDNF) secretion. Thus it appears that the flavonoids may protect against anxiety/depression in asthmatics.

Extracts of the individual ASHMI herbs were tested for potential inhibition of TNF-a production. Of these, *Glycyrrhiza uralensis* produced significant and concentration-dependent inhibition of TNF-a production at all tested concentrations. It happens that *Glycyrrhiza uralensis*, is the herb found in more anti-asthma and mood-disorder formulas than any other. The other two herbs appeared to be less effective.

They focused on whether isoliquiritigen (ILQG) a flavonoid in *Glycyrrhiza uralensis*, inhibits NF-kB activation by measuring p-IkB and IkB levels. NF-kB signaling pathway activation is a necessary step in the production of tumor necrosis factor a (TNF-a), interleukin (IL) 8, and IL-17, which drive neutrophilic inflammation. Pre-treatment of cells with ILQG resulted in reduced p-IkB levels and IkB degradation. In addition to contributing to neurodegenerative process by inducing proinflammatory cytokines, microglia can also induce the release of neurotrophic factors such as BDNF. The authors say, "we observed that pre-treatment with ILQG induced BDNF

---

[44]"Allergic Asthma: When Organ Systems Communicate, We May Not Always Like What They Have to Say," http://asthmaallergieschildren.com/2014/09/06/allergic-asthma-when-organ-systems-communicate-we-may-not-always-like-what-they-have-to-say/

production in a concentration-dependent manner in LPS-stimulated micro-glial cells" What are the effects? They cite a series of other papers on BDNF's effects, including roles in brain health during life and what autopsies of depressed individuals revealed, as well as the anti-depressant effects BDNF infused into the brains of animals. "Ours is the first study to show that treatment of LPS-stimulated microglial cells with ILQG leads to beneficial production of BDNF."

They conclude:

> In this study, we showed that ASHMI and its herbal constituents *Glycyrrhiza uralensis* flavonoids inhibit TNF-a production by LPS stimulated microglial cells and elevate BDNF levels. Further studies are required to fully elucidate the mechanisms of action underlying ASHMI and its compounds CNS anti-inflammatory effects, and to investigate clinical benefit in asthma patients with comorbid anxiety/depression.

As my friend and co-author Dr. Larry Chiaramonte said to me when I showed him evidence of ASHMI's anti-inflammatory effects without concomitant cytotoxicity and mood-related effects, "Sounds like the Holy Grail."

"Bootleg" ASHMI

In the United States, where herbal medicines can be used as supplements even before they are approved as pharmaceuticals, word of ASHMI's effectiveness spread through the alternative medicine community and reached the supplement industry. Thus, Dr. Li became aware at one point that a product had appeared on the market that even used the trademarked name. It is simpler to enforce trademark infringement than it is to enforce patent infringement, and after a cease-and-desist letter, this bootleg version was given a different name, but continued to be sold.

I learned about it when a respectable integrative medicine clinic wrote to Dr. Li asking if she could supply ASHMI for their patients who were using the bootleg version with great success for upper and lower airway inflammation, but was not certified as compliant with California regulations, which are very important because California is such a huge market. Herb toxicity is cited frequently in the organ transplant center at a major university hospital in the State where Chinese medicine is popular, according to friends who work there.

I have also heard from herbalists in other countries about their interest in the drug and their own versions that they use with their patients.

If imitation is the sincerest form of flattery, the spontaneous market for this well-studied, effective drug is an indication at very least of frustration with the mainstream formulary and the desire for something both effective and side effect free. The mothers whose children are receiving treatment in Dr. Li's private practice write regularly about their child going steroid and albuterol free through an entire pollen or cold season.

Maria P — Case Study I

While most of Dr. Li's asthma patients have multiple allergic conditions, the asthma patients who stand out are "chronically steroid dependent. When they are on steroids they still have symptoms."

Maria P. is a 62-year old California woman who was born in pre-Castro Cuba where she experienced her first reaction to a peanut at age two during a visit to the local zoo. The reaction and waking up in the hospital where she was receiving high doses of the steroid decadron are her first memories.

Newly aware of the hazards of peanuts during the remainder of the family's time in Cuba and a couple of years in Spain where they moved as the political situation in Cuba became untenable, she says that avoidance was not that difficult, and she escaped without further incident until at the age of 11 or 12 when she rubbed a peanut on her skin on a dare.

It was not until 1965 when they finally settled in Orange County, California where Maria has lived ever since, that peanuts, peanut products, and other foods became a continual threat. By then, she was also extremely asthmatic as well. She was so reactive that when she fell in love at age 17, the boy's parents sat him down and said, "This girl is so sick — are you sure you want to marry her?" The young couple persisted, and they were married two years later, and they have been married ever since.

The next 30 years were a roller coaster of raising children and reading labels alternating with anaphylaxis and asthma, systemic and inhaled steroids, long courses of antibiotics, avoiding homes with dogs and cats, and hospitalizations. Everywhere they went, they took epinephrine, albuterol, and Benadryl. Even when her symptoms were well controlled, she would wake up in the middle of the night to find that her husband was watching her breathe. When they went out to restaurants, where they would carefully interrogate waiters, managers, and chefs about the potential for allergen contamination, her ever-loyal husband would not touch his food until she had tasted hers. In Southern California, where the legendary Santa Ana winds rage, often accompanied by wildfires, even non-asthmatics avoid going outside; Maria would remain sealed in her home with the air-conditioning on.

She wrote recently,

> I was constantly using my rescue inhaler, I had a portable breathing machine with me and I was on high levels of steroids. I was also using either Advair then I was switched to Pulmicort. I have been hospitalized if I came down with a simple cold. During the spring months my allergies went into a frenzy. I was addicted to nose drops.

Given the limitations, the P. family has lived a remarkably adventurous and travel-filled life, punctuated by a few near misses, like the anaphylaxis that Maria suffered while visiting her son at singing camp, and another during a cruise when the chef neglected to connect her careful instructions with his recipe for chocolate mousse. Fortunately for her, the ship's doctor had recently lost a close friend to anaphylaxis and was hyper-aware of the treatment protocols.

The long-term toll on Maria's health was considerable. She had diminished lung function. She had extreme weight gain during prolonged treatment with prednisone and antibiotics with mood swings to match. (Systemic steroid use causes patients to retain water, eat more, and move less because of discomfort from chronic inflammation. It also tends to redistribute fat, which accounts for the characteristic "moon face.") Her doctor told her that if she could see her lungs, they would be strawberry red from inflammation. She and her husband were continually on the lookout for new treatments, and that led them to Mount Sinai where there was an early clinical trial of one of Dr. Li's ASHMI. While she was turned down for falling outside the subject profile, Dr. Li told her that she could treat her as a private patient.

The early treatment involved 90 pills a day, including food allergy treatments, immune boosters, and metabolism boosters.

Maria writes,

> After visiting Dr. Li and starting my Chinese teas, gradually I began to feel
> better. The first six months there was a slight improvement, although I was
> on high doses of the teas. As the first year came around I started getting
> off my oral steroids and stayed on Advair. I got off all asthma medications
> a year into my program, although I still carry my rescue inhaler and I have
> a full supply of antibiotics in case I get sick during my travels.

Maria has had intermittent non-related issues. During preparation for and
rehab from orthopedic surgery, she took a four-month hiatus from the
herbal treatment, with no relapse. Pulmonary function was 114% of normal,
compared to 80% pre-treatment.

She writes,

> I have followed Dr. Li's advice in working close to my internist. I've had
> the flu twice and I told my husband, "I'm like a regular person, fever, head-
> ache, body ache, but NO ASTHMA." My internist always puts me on
> antibiotics when I get the flu to keep me from getting bronchitis, and my
> doctor is thrilled with my progress.

She is now down to 10 pills, twice a day.

Finally, Maria has managed to lose 60 pounds.

> I can't even think back [to] when I was so ill I could hardly function. I am
> able to do so many things I never imagined. I dance, I go boating, I travel
> to places I never could have dreamed of going due to my constantly being
> short of breath. I sometimes forget that I ever had asthma. I am no longer
> swollen like a balloon from all the steroids, local and oral. Overall I have
> never felt better and been in such good health.

Are these gains permanent? As Dr. Li says,

> They got better on the herbs and eventually they were off all inhaled ster-
> oids. In these cases they stop the herbs for six months and go back on
> herbs for six months — that is the protocol. Most of the time I start with
> a one-month alternating protocol. Maybe eventually they will only need
> three months treatment per year. I am happy when they are able to wean

off the steroids, but I am also happy when they can stop TCM when their conditions are well controlled.

"Donna" — Case Study II

One year after "Donna" began treatment with Dr. Li, her mother reported with excitement that her peanut IgE had gone from 83.9 to 43.8, almost 50% improvement, that her tree nut IgE had fallen almost to nothing, and most important that her asthma was under control. Donna a college student, reports,

> I have had pretty bad asthma since I was a kid. Before starting the herbs, I was on four different daily medications to control my asthma. Now, I am off of all of them, I only have a rescue inhaler, which I need about once a week. After about five months being on the herbs, I was able to run on the treadmill a couple times a week, and that's something I've never been able to do!

Her mother adds,

> Regarding the asthma, every cold meant inhaler, nebulizer, and hope that we could make it through the night without a trip to the ER. There were times I just wanted to breathe for her or count the seconds between coughing fits.... she was very fortunate to have a gym teacher in elementary school who was aware and kind, but things like sports and playing the clarinet took too much air. We live in a mountainous area so we're short on the O_2 anyway.
>
> After we started this treatment and she told me that she started running on a treadmill or hiking in the mountains, I was panicked. Then on one of the school breaks she said casually she was no longer on one of the inhalers and was thinking about stopping other stuff. We were so excited, but scared!!! The nuts/peanuts is amazing but it always seemed like asthma stood in her way and I think with this treatment her lungs are healing or figuring out how to work better!!

Chapter

3

ATOPIC DERMATITIS

My conversations with Dr. Li started with atopic dermatitis (AD or eczema). She told me that her offsite clinic began with it. Other doctors would send her what she calls their "give-up" patients, those whose skin was untreatable by the best that Western medicine had to throw at them, and which was so bad day-to-day that it often made life almost unbearable. She chose to start with AD in private practice because the protocols could be administered simultaneously with steroids and other treatments, which could then be tapered off safely as skin very visibly showed improvement.

Atopic dermatitis is another allergic disease I have active sympathy with. My late mother told me I had it when I was a baby, although for some reason I do not have any memory of that. Allergic rhinitis and asthma followed in time. However, I currently have a condition called spongiotic dermatitis, which showed up a few years ago. SD has one important symptom in common with AD — the urge to treat the afflicted tissue with sandpaper.

People will go to great lengths to achieve some relief, even at the expense of their own long-term health. While most people are wary of steroids and will avoid their use even when it is really bad for them, which happens often with asthma, AD patients will use them too much. Pediatric dermatologist, Dr. James Treat of the University of Pennsylvania says that many patients, particularly teenage girls, will use the strongest medicines if it is the only thing that gives them relief and then persist to the point where their skin is dangerously thin and their immune systems are weak. My cousin, pediatric allergist Dr. Paul Ehrlich, calls me in a state of semi-despair now and then because a new patient has been describing her thoughts of suicide over the painful state of her skin. He recalls that when he was a pediatric resident at Bellevue Hospital in the 1970s, children admitted with severe eczema were tied down to keep them from scratching while being dosed with antihistamines.

AD is considered the first step in the "atopic march." That is, the first indication other than family history that a child is disposed to allergies, and is often followed by some combination of environmental allergies, asthma, and food allergies. The skin fails in its role as the primary defense against the outside world, leaving patients vulnerable to a range of antigens — microbes, viruses, and allergens.

The possible role of the skin as the starting point for allergic sensitization has been drawing more and more attention, particularly to foods, and especially for peanut. British researchers have found that peanut residue is stubborn and biologically active in homes where lots of peanut products are consumed. Eczematous skin is vulnerable to these residues, which can penetrate in sufficient quantities to start an immune response.[45]

According to an update of practice parameters written by dermatologist Peter Lio and others, "AD is associated with impaired skin barrier function, a proinflamammatory atopic response to antigens, and reduced cutaneous antimicrobial activity" whose "molecular pathways interact and potentiate each other" necessitating treatment for all three. Understanding of skin-barrier dysfunction leapt forward in 2006 with the discovery of filaggrin gene (FLG) mutations.[46]

Like asthma, AD is hard to diagnose. Dr. Lio and his colleagues point to

a constellation of clinical features, which include pruritus and chronic or relapsing eczematous lesions with typical morphology and distribution...

---

[45] Helen Brough, et al., "Peanut protein in household dust is related to household peanut consumption and is biologically active," Journal of Allergy and Clinical Immunology September 2013; 132(3): 630–638.

[46] Peter A. Lio, "An Overview of Atopic Dermatitis Diagnosis," Practical Dermatology April 2014; http://practicaldermatology.com/2014/04/an-overview-of-atopic-dermatitis-diagnosis/

The distribution of AD can vary with age as well as with disease activity. In younger children and infants, the scalp, face, neck, and extensor surfaces of the skin are often involved. In older children and adults, flexural areas are more commonly seen with lichenification, thickening, in addition to acute inflammatory changes.

Other conditions that mimic AD and must be ruled out are scabies, seborrheic dermatitis, contact dermatitis, ichthyoses, cutaneous T-cell lymphoma, and psoriasis.

Patients are continually looking for alternatives and adjuncts for the allergy treatment, hydration, and steroids that represent standard care. Dr. Lio wrote a review of current options being explored for the website I edit.[47]

One was the use of silk to augment cotton in kids' clothing, citing a 2007 study that compared children wearing silk with a special coating around their elbows (like knees, elbows are eczema prone) to a control group wearing only cotton.

> The experimental group did consistently better at weeks 4, 8, and 12. Silk is hypothesized to aid wound healing by enhancing collagen synthesis and reducing edema and inflammation; this specially coated silk also has antimicrobial properties, which is significant since the skin normally has staphylococcus aureus (staph) germs sitting on it that can penetrate when scratched and cause infections, and may fuel inflammation by its very presence.

Another textile candidate is silver coating, which also has an anti-bacterial effect.

Climate and humidity also influence eczema. One study moved patients from subarctic/temperate Norway to sunny subtropical Gran Canary, and their skin improved compared to controls. Another involved whole-body cooling (cryotherapy) at temperatures down to $-110°C$ (166°F) three times a week. Peter wrote, "The authors suggested that the effect was related to reduced nerve conduction velocity and decreased synthesis of acetylcholine in the nerve ganglia, both of which could influence itch." It is hard to picture

---

[47] Peter A. Lio, "Beyond Medications: Treatments for Atopic Dermatitis," January 2014; http://asthmaallergieschildren.com/2014/01/01/beyond-medications-treatments-for-atopic-dermatitis/

this as a mass treatment, although "using water-filled passive cooling" bedding has shown some promise.

Other experiments have involved therapeutic bathing at such ancient sites as the Dead Sea, and French and Italian springs that were popular with armies during the Roman Empire, and probably before that.

Clearly, the patient population is open to new possibilities.

Suffering by the Numbers

The misery of AD is evaluated on various subjective scales. One is called the SCORAD index that "combines body surface area measurements with signs of intensity, and symptoms of itch and sleeplessness, to calculate a score of 0–103 for disease severity." [48]

The sites affected by eczema are shaded on a drawing of a body. The rule of nine is used to calculate the affected area (A) as a percentage of the whole body.

Head and neck 9%
Upper limbs 9% each
Lower limbs 18% each
Anterior trunk 18%
Back 18%
1% for genitals

The score for each area is added up. The total area is 'A', which has a possible maximum of 100%.

Intensity

A representative area of eczema is selected. In this area, the intensity of each of the following signs is assessed as none (0), mild (1), moderate (2) or severe (3).

Redness
Swelling
Oozing/crusting

---

[48] http://www.dermnetnz.org/dermatitis/scorad.html

Scratch marks

Skin thickening (lichenification)

Dryness (this is assessed in an area where there is no inflammation)

Another measure is the Dermatology Quality of Life Index (DQLI), ten questions that help assess the impact of the disease on a scale from 0 to 30. The questions not only encompass physical symptoms, such as pain and itching, but also behavior, choice of wardrobe, and social and sexual activity. I took this test after 5 bi-weekly appointments with a dermatologist who painted me with liquid nitrogen in addition to use of topical steroids and moisturizers. At that point I scored an 8.

If I had taken the DQLI before treatment, I would undoubtedly have done worse, but not nearly as bad as badly as 14 patients, ages 6 months to 52 years old with a median age of 5.4 years, treated by Dr. Li and written up in a 2015 paper written by a team headed by Julia A. Wisniewski, MD. In that study, the baseline levels ranged from 10 to 30, with a median score of 17. The SCORAD index showed a range from 42–103, with a median of 89, and 13 out of 14 were above 50 (published as abstract).[49]

These patients were chosen through retrospective analysis of all who had been treated for eczema at Dr. Li's clinic between August 2006 and May 2008 in accordance with standards from the Mount Sinai Hospital Review Board. Patients were instructed to continue or discontinue previously instituted treatments for eczema at the discretion of their referring physicians. Use of concurrent eczema treatments was recorded in the chart at the time of starting TCM and discontinuation of medications was recorded at follow-up visits. Each patient chart was reviewed for demographic information, then reviewed about once a month to assess how careful subjects were maintaining their TCM regimen, conventional medication use, SCORAD, DQLI index, results of routine safety results like kidney and liver function, and total and specific IgE values.

Previous experiments for eczema with TCM by other researchers centered on a ten-herb mixture investigated under the name Zemaphyte. The herbs are traditionally simmered as tea for 90 minutes and drunk. It was

---

[49] J. Wisniewski, A. Nowak-Wegrzyn, E. Steenburgh-Thanik, H. Sampson, X. Li, "efficacy and safety of traditional chinese medicine for treatment of atopic dermatitis (AD)," *Journal of Allergy and Clinical Immunology* February 2009; 123(2), Supplement: S37.

found to be generally successful at reducing itching and improving sleep, but was accompanied in some cases by adverse effects that included gastrointestinal upset, urticaria, photosensitivity, exacerbation of eczema, night diuresis, discoloration of teeth, and elevated liver enzymes and creatinine levels. Two children also developed liver-function abnormalities. All these side effects normalized after discontinuation of treatment.

For Dr. Li's 14-patient study, median patient age was 5.4 years, ranging in age from 6 months to 52 years, including 9 males and 5 females. In addition to the alarming SCORAD profile, other measures were also very high. Only 12 of the subjects had been tested for total IgE — the sum of all the allergic antibodies found in a volume of blood — but the median baseline for total IgE for them was 4,545, ranging from 95–37,390. Eczema had started in infancy in all cases, including the 52-year old, and half of them started before two months. Median disease duration prior to starting TCM was 40 months, but one child had been suffering continuously for 14 years. The adult had suffered for his entire life. Caucasians comprised 57% of the study population with one Hispanic patient and four of Southeast Asian background. All patients had family histories of atopy in a 1st degree relative — parent or sibling. The youngest patient had only atopic dermatitis. The other 13 had other allergic diseases in various combinations; four had asthma, four had allergic rhinitis, and many had environmental allergies. All 13 of these patients reported food allergies: 10 had confirmed allergies to milk, 13 to egg, 9 to soy, 10 to wheat, 12 to peanut, 3 to fish, and 1 patient carried a diagnosis of Food Protein-Induced Enterocolitis Syndrome [FPIES]. Environment allergies were to dogs (6 patients), cats (5), dust (1), molds (8), and tree pollens (7). Other co-morbid illness included poor weight gain, anxiety, depression, and frequent stomachaches.

The Treatment

There were three avenues of therapy: an internal remedy, several external compounds, and acupuncture. To test their safety, the herbal preparations were fed to mice at levels 24 times the human doses with no adverse effects.

Internal Remedy: Erka Shi Zhen Herbal Tea, in practice called *Shi Zhen* tea, an extract of nine herbs (10g/bag, produced by Xiyuan Chinese Medicine Research and Pharmaceutical Manufacturer, Xiyuan Hospital, China Academy of Traditional Chinese Medicine Science, Beijing, China 100091 — a GPP facility equivalent to GMP facility), imported under FDA guidelines as a dietary supplement (FDA registration #: 13448111832). All raw herbs had met standards of the Pharmacopoeia of the People's Republic of China (Vol. 1, 2000). Contents of heavy metals, pesticides, and microbials met all FDA guidelines.

Effect of TCM in Infant/Young Children Eczema

	Age	sex		Onset age	SCORAD Before and during of TCM				Skin lesion improvement Of TCM (%)		
					0	1 M	3 M	6 M	1 M	3 M	6 M
P1	6 M	M	White	3w	80.9	24.2	3.7	0	60	90	100
P2	8M	M	White	6 m	70.5	5.3	0	NA	70	100	NA
P3	12M	M	White	3m	65.3	NA	NA	4	70	80	95
P4	16M	M	Asian	3m	69	14.3	0	0	60	80	100
P5	17M	F	White	1w	101	13.5	0	0	50	100	100
P6	36M	F	White	24m	45	0	0	0	100	100	100
P7	36M	F	White/black	3m	56	14.3	0	0	60	100	100
P8	4Y	M	White	2w	83.4	22.7	9.0	1.8	50	80	100
P9	17	F	White	1w	50	15.2	0	0	50	100	100
P10	7m	M	White	7m	10.7	0	0	0	100	100	100

The tea was prescribed for a first day schedule of one packet of tea dissolved in boiling water (approximately 50 mL) in the morning, then waiting for 10–15 minutes before drinking only 2 teaspoons of tea. During the next 24 hours the patient was to be monitored for adverse reactions. On the second day and thereafter, one packet of tea was prepared in the same way, twice a day and drunk.

External Remedies: Bath additive containing eight individually extracted herbs. The patient soaked in the bath with herbs for 20–30 minutes a day. Herbal cream containing two herbs made at the China-Japan Friendship Hospital in Beijing was applied to the skin, 2–3 times a day. Acupaste made from two grams of FAHF-2[50] powder (Xiyuan Chinese Medicine Research and Pharmaceutical Manufacturer, Xiyuan Hospital, China Academy of Traditional Chinese Medicine Science, Beijing, China) was prescribed. The

---

[50] Food Allergy Herbal Formula-2, a nine-herb compound developed to treat food allergies and a NIH/NCCAM registered investigational drug.

powder was mixed with water and the paste was applied to an acupoint, *Shen Que* (belly button), which was changed daily. The acupaste was omitted for patients with open lesions until they healed.

Acupuncture at the *Zu San Li* and *Qu Chi* acupoints was recommended approximately every two weeks.

Results

Medication Use

Half the patients had been treated intermittently with oral corticosteroids before starting TCM treatment, including five who had taken oral steroids in the previous three months. Three months after therapy began, oral steroid use fell by 25%. All patients reported topical steroids on-and-off, including half of the 14 patients in the three months prior to presentation. Topical steroid use went down by 21% after three months. The reduction in both oral and topical steroid use after three months was 29%. Antihistamines, which all patients used, including 11 out of 14 at the onset of TCM, were reduced by 32% after three months.

Effect of TCM on Infant/Young Children
Eczema: Reduction of Steroid Use

	Age	sex	Onset	Steroid use before and during TCM			
	M			0M	1M	3M	6m
P1	6	M	3w	200 (2.5%HCx2)	50 (1%HCx1)	1%	0%
P2	8	M	6 m	200 (2.5%HCx2)	50 (1%HCx1)	0	NA
P3	12	M	3m	300 (Triam.x1)	200 2.5%HC	100 (1% HC)	5% (1% HC)
P4	16	M	3m	300 (Flut.x1)	100-50 (1%HCx1)	0	0
P5	17	F	1w	0	0	0	0
P6	36	F	24m	300 (Triama.x1)	150 (Triam. erd)	100 (1% HC)	10 (1% HC)
P7	36	F	3m	300 (Desonide)	50	0	0
P8	48	M	2w	400 (pred. 8d/m)	0	0	0
P9	17	F	1w	150 (protopic)	0	0	0
P10	7	M	7m	0	0	0	0

Three patients had used stronger immune suppressants, such as cyclosporine, although only one was doing so at the time of starting TCM; this was discontinued by the three month mark. Five patients had tried other types of alternative therapies prior to their referral for TCM. While all patients reported histories of food allergy, only 10 of the 14 of patients reported managing their eczema by avoiding foods. Some foods were successfully reintroduced over the study period, but no patient was able to follow a completely unrestricted diet.

Quality of Life

Quality of life improved measured by both SCORAD and DQLI. During the first three months of treatment, seven patients experienced 60–90% improvement (classified as "good"), and sustained it over 15 months of follow-up. One patient achieved excellent improvement (>90%) in the first three months, which was sustained for 5.4 months, the last report before the study was written up. Seven patients showed inadequate (<60%) improvement in SCORAD in the first 1–3 months, but attained good or excellent improvement over the following 3–15 months. At the end of the study period, 12 patients had sustained good (>60%) improvement, and five out of 14 had sustained excellent improvement (>90%). Improved quality of life, especially improvements in sleep and pruritus, were observed sooner than improvements in skin quality and SCORAD. Eleven of 14 patients experienced at least a 50% improvement in quality of life during the first 1–3 months of therapy. At the end of the study period, 12 of 14 patients reported sustained improvement in quality of life with ten of 14 reporting >80% improvement.

All patients tolerated TCM treatment well. No one stopped using the medications due to side effects. There were no episodes of staphyloccus. Staph aureus germs often sit on the surface of the skin where they probably exert some protective effect as part of the skin microbiome, but can cause infections if introduced into sublayers of the skin with scratching or through lesions. Nor were there other infections in any patients during the follow-up period. There was no documented anemia, leucopenia, thrombocytopenia, liver enzyme elevation, or renal dysfunction.

Peripheral eosinophilia decreased from $1,000 \pm 700$ mc/L to 500 ± 200 (P = 0.03) with no change in total blood counts. Baseline total IgE was available for 12 of 14 patients (see page 9) and subsequent total IgE values were available for ten of those 12 patients. A decreasing trend in total IgE was observed in seven patients, and an increasing trend in total IgE in 2.

These outcomes were noteworthy for many reasons, particularly since high IgE at baseline has been described as a predictor of poor response to conventional treatment for AD. Two patients in this group had begun at 16,892 and 21,135, and, as mentioned, 37,390.[51]

Treating anyone for the painful and demoralizing experience of recalcitrant eczema makes the world a better place, even if the relief is temporary, as with steroids. To these patients, the prospect of longer-term relief without side effects — well, that sounds like a blessing. Slowing the atopic march and sparing small children a lifetime of chronic allergic disease sounds like a miracle. But how to bring these promising benefits to a wider patient population?

Building a Network of Practitioners

In my other book I talked about the problem of extending Dr. Li's methods and medications beyond her one day a week solo practice, and monthly follow-up phone conversations. She sketched a program for mentoring mainstream practitioners to use her medicines, and to create what she calls a "practice network." After publication, a West Coast allergist wrote to Dr. Li to ask if he could learn to use her methods.

In 2015, I helped Dr. Li organize a seminar to educate allopathic allergists to use her medicines to treat their patients. Held in July, this was the first stab at building a practice network to expand the use of these medicines without necessarily teaching the theory and vocabulary of TCM.

As we discussed that day, the target parameters for these patients start at daily use of topical steroids of 2.5% — two and a half times the strongest over-the-counter medications. These medicines are powerful enough to thin the skin and compromise the immune system if they are used for too long.

---

[51] V. Kiiski, O. Karlsson, A, Remitz, S. Reitamo, "High serum total IgE predicts poor long-term outcome in atopic dermatitis," *Acta Dermata-Venereologica*; http://www.medicaljournals.se/acta/content/?doi=10.2340/00015555-2126&html=1

At the upper end, these patients use systemic steroids as often as 8 days per month. People who use steroids at these levels are desperate for relief.

The regimen includes three types of herbal cream. The first of these are to be administered at the initial, most acute stages, when there are open sores. It can go right on the lesions. The second is during the recovery phase. The third is for recovered skin to maintain the earlier gains; this can also be used as a sunscreen.

There is a herbal bath additive.

Finally, there are three internal teas, one for acute eczema, one for excessive, irresistible itching that do not respond to antihistamines, and a third for chronic eczema.

Looking down the list of herbal ingredients and their applications for treating other diseases, one begins to get a feel for the synergy that makes these particular combinations useful for treating eczema.

For example, *yin hua*, or *flos lonicerae Joponica*, is used in TCM to treat skin infections such as carbuncles and mastitis but also the flu and pneumonia, and even appendicitis. It has anti-bacterial, anti-viral, and anti-inflammatory properties.

Qing dai, folium isatidis, is an anti-bacterial that has been used to treat upper respiratory infections, measles, and pneumonia.

Zi cao, radix arnebiae seu Lithospermi, is anti-bacterial, analgesic, and anti-inflammatory. It promotes regeneration of the epidermis and has been used to treat burns and psoriasis.

Other herbs have anti-fungal properties.

During the session, one of the doctors raised the issue of bowel movements as therapy progressed. This was news to me, but apparently both diarrhea and constipation accompany severe eczema. Curious about this, I inquired from my social network of patient mothers what their experience had been. Sure enough, many reported significant improvements both in the too-much and too-little categories of bowel disturbance. Clues to this resolution are buried not-too-deeply in the data on the different herbs, which are described variously as treatments for indigestion, "food stagnation", and diarrhea. Significantly for anyone who has lain awake scratching, there is something called *fu ling*, which treats insomnia as well as diarrhea and edema.[52]

---

[52] http://www.tcmwiki.com/wiki/fu-ling

All of these herbs are not only employed in routine treatment of various conditions not connected to eczema, per se, but they have been studied for their mechanisms of action that are pertinent to their effects on the skin. For example, *lin qiao* (Fructus forsythia suspensae) can be used as an anti-bacterial against staph aureus, among many other microbes, which, as stated earlier, often sits on the skin and can cause infections when dug in by scratching. It also has anti-viral and anti-inflammatory uses.

Fortunately, the allopathic doctors who will one day use these compounds for their oozing, suffering patients do not have to know all of that. The acute creams are formulated either for very dry lesions and very wet ones, and they can be alternated as conditions change.

Dr. Li informed us that adapting traditional formulations to the full spectrum of allergic patients is complicated by the range of allergies. For example, sesame oil is the best medium for mixing the herbs for uptake and pliability, but sesame is a major allergen, and with constant use on damaged skin, there is a possibility of sensitization. Cornstarch and corn oil are useful because they are substantially protein free, but they may affect those with mast cell problems that are not IgE mediated.

The presentation culminated in a series of case histories of small children who registered dramatic improvements as measured by healing of skin lesions, diminished use of steroids, and enhanced quality of life. One was a 19-month-old boy with chronic and unremitting eczema since three months of age with allergies to 25 foods tested, and avoidance diet for egg, milk, wheat, soy, oat, barley, rye, peanuts, tree nuts, fish, shellfish, seeds, legumes, chicken, lamb, garlic, broccoli, apple, and raspberry. After two months, his eczematous lesions improved by 80%. After 5–6 months of treatment, there were no eczematous lesions. Surprisingly, total serum IgE reduced from 4091 to 749 kIU/L, 17 food-specific IgE levels were reduced by 40% to 80%.

Another was an eight-year old boy referred by a pediatric allergist who had suffered with eczema since he was a baby, despite the use of high-potency topical steroids. He, too, had many food and environmental allergies.

After therapy consisting of acupressure and then acupuncture (every 2–4 weeks), herbal formulas (15 capsules, twice a day), herbal cream, (twice a day) and herbal bath (once a day) more than 80% of his skin improved within 4–6 months while switching from high potency to OTC 1%

hydrocortisone, and almost 90–100% improvement at 12 months; and 100% improvement at 1½years. His total and specific IgE also improved. He continues his treatment for his food allergy.

Reducing IgE to Specific Foods While Treating the Skin

As the semi-official social-media contact person for Dr. Li's patients, patients' parents, and those who are considering her treatment, one of the questions I see regularly is "which medicine does what?" in a treatment program that encompasses multiple allergic conditions. The answer is that the medicines act in concert involving multiple organ systems that may variously affect the skin, the lungs, and so forth. Since 40% of severely eczematous patients also have food and other allergies, achieving relief for the skin also entails moderating other allergic mechanisms. The patients described above achieved dramatic lowering of total and specific IgE. Jackie O, a girl whom I wrote about in my first book, saw her total IgE fall from 6,000 to about 500 kU/L (thousand units per liter).

At the 2015 convention of the American Academy of Allergy, Asthma and Immunology (AAAAI), Dr. Li's team presented data on one of the topical treatments in the anti-eczema regime on peanut-specific IgE. This is the antibody that epitomizes the food allergy epidemic. It is the stand-in for the fears and hopes of millions of families. The researchers are studying different components of the herbal treatments to isolate the exact means that will prove most productive as they strive for ever-more-efficient dosing regimes.[53,54]

Berberine and indigo *naturalis* extracts, which are known to suppress IgE production in a human B cell line, are active ingredients in Herbal Cream

---

[53]Chaoyi Mao, MD; Ying Song, MD; Zhenwen Zhou, PhD; Changda Liu, PhD; Kamal D. Srivastava, PhD; Farid Jahouh, PhD; Rong Wang, PhD; Xiaoping Yan; Xiu-Min Li, MD, "Acute anti-IgE effect of topical application of formulation of herbal extracts in a peanut allergic murine model," *Journal of Allergy and Clinical Immunology* February 2015; 135(2), Supplement: AB29.

[54]Nan Yang, Julie Wang, Changda Liu, Ying Song, Shuwei Zhang, Jiachen Zi, Jixun Zhan, Madhan Masilamani *et al.*, "Berberine and limonin suppress IgE production by human B cells and peripheral blood mononuclear cells from food-allergic patients," *Annals of Allergy, Asthma and Immunology* 2014; 113(5): 556–564.e4.

III-B. It was rubbed into a set of peanut-sensitized mice at various intervals, with a set of sham-treated mice as a control. Sera were obtained one day prior to and one day after treatment, total and peanut specific antibodies were measured by ELISA, as were IL-4, IL-10 and IFN-γ production by cultured mesenteric lymph node (MLN) cells and splenocytes, which means there was no loss of these protective cytokines. Berberine absorption in serum was also measured.

The cream was shown to decrease serum peanut-specific IgE and total IgE levels by 78% and 52% respectively compared to baseline (p < 0.001 for both), with no significant changes in peanut specific and total IgE levels before and after sham treatment. MLN cells and splenocytes from Herbal-Cream-IIIb treated mice showed no significant difference in peanut protein induced IL-4, IL-10 and IFN-γ production compared to MLN cells and splenocytes from sham treated mice. Serum berberine concentrations peaked one hour following topical application. The upshot of this is that the cream may be a useful adjunct for peanut allergy treatment even without eczema. Moreover, further study with other allergens may also show improvement, since there was nothing specific to peanut in the actual treatment.

Dosing is a Compliance Issue

As with FAHF-2, the daily intake of pills is a barrier to effectiveness. A full dose of *Shi Zhen* tea is 15 pills twice a day. Based on the experience with butanol extraction to transform FAHF-2 into the much more concentrated B-FAHF-2, Dr. Li's lab has started to apply this technology to *Shi Zhen*. The topical treatments have compliance issues of their own. The creams initially tint skin different colors. The smallest children are the easiest to treat not only because their immune systems are malleable, but also because they do not worry about turning green temporarily. Also, clothing and bedding may require more rapid than normal replacement, because the medicines stain. But there is no getting around diligent treatment. As one mother points out, it is not like flossing before a dentist appointment.

"Sally G"

For the first 18 months of her life, Sally's eczema was "horrible." It reached a low point at Thanksgiving in 2013 when visiting her grandma and grandpa in upstate New York. The air was exceptionally dry, both outdoors where it was very cold and indoors where it was warm. Her shoulders and upper back were so damaged that they stuck to her clothes when she was undressed and skin peeled off.

According to Susan, Sally's mother, her little girl was born with perfect skin, but at just three days old, she began to break out in hives. Susan, admitting to wishful thinking that it would go away, tried to overlook them in hopes that they would clear up on their own. She would take pictures on what she remembers as "good days" but in reviewing those pictures, they did not look so good. She realizes now that her standards changed. Bad days were so bad that "less-bad" days would look good enough to photograph.

The pediatrician said it was the most dramatic case she had seen. Still, Sally had a good appetite and slept well, although her scratching was so fierce that she had to be dressed in long sleeves and turtlenecks even when the weather was warm. Topical steroids and wet wraps became nightly features.

Susan had worked in finance and was an expert researcher. She came across Dr. Li's name in December 2013, the month after the disastrous Thanksgiving.

Through blood test results, Dr. Li learned that Sally was allergic to milk, eggs, nuts, and a longer list of things.

Dr. Li explained that children with eczema are more likely to develop asthma. And that staying on the treatment program until Sally is five years old would best position her to stave off asthma.

Sally was put on a regimen of three herbal medicines, *Shi Zhen* teas, *Shi Zhen* creams, and digestive tea. Initially, the cream stained her skin black because of the ingredients, but Dr. Li said that as her skin healed the discoloration would decrease, which proved to be the case. Office visits also involved a short session of massage.

Within a month, there was pronounced improvement, and by six months, there was a single "rough patch" on Sally's right wrist and no "red dots." Now, more than a year after commencing treatment, Sally usually has perfect-looking skin.

"Megan C"

Megan, now aged four, was born with food allergies. She showed allergy to dairy at three days old when she projectile vomited after her mother, Andrea, ate cottage cheese and breastfed her after that. With time they learned she was also allergic to eggs, peanuts and tree nuts. She also had GI issues; a few times as a toddler, she had 4–8 week bouts of stubborn diarrhea following administration of an antibiotic for pneumonia at seven months.

She always had mild eczema but Andrea could usually manage it with coconut oil or occasional over-the-counter hydrocortisone. She passed the skin and blood tests, and food challenges for eggs and peanuts, so those were incorporated into her diet. At age 2½, her eczema began to get gradually worse. Her allergist re-did her skin test and found a reaction to peanuts, so that was removed from her diet. Sadly, it did not help the eczema, which within a couple of months had spread everywhere below her neck.

Life at Age 3

Megan scratched constantly, which made her eczema worse. Andrea says,

> We couldn't get the scratching under control. She was on Claritin and Benadryl every single day, and it helped only slightly. She was also using prescription steroids. At first using it just 50% of the time (which is what our pediatrician recommended) and that kept it under control. With time we had to use it more and more though, and even when [we] got to using it 100% of the time, the eczema was still there.
>
> Last summer poor Megan looked like she had chicken pox and strangers would stop us on the street to ask if she had some type of disease. She looked miserable with red, itchy, broken skin and Band-Aids everywhere to try to keep her from scratching the most broken skin. She was a very unhappy, emotional child.
>
> Sleep was absolutely horrible for my husband, me, and my daughter. She was awake many times in the night, crying because her skin hurt [from the] incessant itching. Her sheets were bloody every morning from the broken skin that she kept scratching. I tried putting socks on her hands at night but she would cry so hard and rip them off immediately. She got to the point of not being able to wear shoes because the eczema was so bad on the tops of her feet. She went barefoot for a week.

She tested positive for bacterial infection on her skin, but with an early history of reaction to antibiotics that had led to eight weeks of diarrhea, her allergist told them to make every effort to stop the scratching before resorting to antibiotics. The parents wet wrapped her twice a day, an old therapy that hydrates dry, permeable skin and protects it from little fingernails.

Wet-wrapping is very time consuming.

> She would take a bath for 10–20 minutes. She would get out and we put prescription steroid on her skin. We then put tight pajamas on her and put her back in the water to get her completely wet. We then put heavy pajamas on top of her to seal in the moisture of the wet pajamas. We did it as long as she could stand it, from 20 minutes to 2 hours, and then took both pairs of pajamas off. Then we put Vaniply on all over her body and put her in real clothes. We did this twice a day. She would cry the entire time she had to be in wet pajamas. It did help tremendously though and was the fastest quick fix for bad flare-ups.

The parents also allowed her to sleep with them. Says Andrea, "I would wake her up several times a night when I heard her scratching, and she would stop so she could stay sleeping next to me. Thankfully, this stopped the scratching and her breaking open even more places on her skin."

Her skin improved but always teetered on the edge of major flares. She would erupt and the parents could not figure out why.

> We worked with a naturopath because even her allergist said there was nothing else she could do for her. We had her on an even more restrictive diet by the suggestion of her naturopath: no gluten, no corn or corn-derived products, and none of her known allergens obviously (dairy, peanuts, tree nuts). We also cut out all nightshades (tomatoes, potatoes, peppers) because they are inflammatory. All of these things helped, but we were on the hunt for a permanent fix for her because she was just headed down a bad path of being more sensitive to more and more foods. We were also just managing the eczema, not curing it. I was desperately reading everything I could to find something to help her and stumbled across Dr. Li's name online. I read as much as I could about her and her work and knew in my heart that this was the answer and the best chance we had of healing our babies.

In November 2014 they started TCM treatment with Dr. Li.

Six Months Later (June 2015)

Her skin is absolutely beautiful and so soft! Friends who have not seen her since last summer comment on how wonderful she looks. She is so much happier, which is no surprise! She tells us how happy she is that "her 'itchies' have gone away". She still has scars from her eczema when it was at its worst, but she does not have any visible red skin or eczema patches anymore.

The first thing we noticed after starting TCM treatment is that she can stand warmer baths. For the prior year, she would always say the water was too hot even though it was lukewarm. (Knowing what I know now, I realize her body was too hot and her skin was burning!) Within a month of starting TCM, she was asking for warmer water.

Now she uses no more prescription steroid whatsoever. She does use 1% hydrocortisone only a few days a week and we are working on getting rid of that completely. This is part of our treatment protocol with Dr. Li.

She still gets random hives sometimes, but the occurrences are much less frequent. We have to be very careful kissing her because if we eat anything she is allergic to, she gets hives. She even gets hives if we put on chapstick and then kiss her. If she even touches a napkin that has uncooked dairy on it, she gets hives.

Sleep is still a major issue in our house, unfortunately. My daughter sleeps in her own bed but because she slept with us for so long to cure her from scratching all night long, she is very dependent on sleeping next to somebody else. She used to be a great sleeper before her eczema got bad, but we have never gotten back to that point.

We are ever-so-gradually adding things back into her diet. She eats nightshades again, and a few times a week we give her products with gluten. She has had no reaction in her skin or GI tract, which is awesome! Recently, due to a mix-up of plates at a restaurant, she ate eggs with butter in them and had no reaction, so we know her dairy allergy is getting better.

Five months after starting TCM treatment, we got blood results for both kids. The total IgE decreased by 1/3 for both of them! With the individual allergens, 90% of my daughter's decreased, and some of them decreased significantly. The others stayed the same or went up. We know what we are doing is working and we will keep on, being 100% complaint with the TCM protocol so we can do our part in healing them the best we can.

4

INFLAMMATORY BOWEL DISEASE

In the previous book, I wrote about David Dunkin, a pediatric gastroenter-ologist at Mount Sinai who works mainly with young patients suffering from inflammatory bowel disease (IBD), such as Crohn's disease (CD) and ulcerative colitis (UC). These are immune-mediated diseases that share symptoms — abdominal pain, rectal bleeding, diarrhea, weight loss, fever, and joint, skin and eye involvement. In addition, when clinicians have trouble distinguishing between them, they use the term "indeterminate colitis" and "IBD undetermined" in referring to it. In Crohn's disease, which was studied and named at Mount Sinai by Dr. Burrill Bernard Crohn in 1932, there can be damage from the mouth to the anus. Genetics play a large part in causing IBD, with large numbers of genes involved, but environmental and dietary factors also play a large part in children. (Tobacco use is also a major factor for adults.) IBD is also driven by "disturbances in the innate and acquired immune systems."[55]

Dr. Dunkin says that Crohn's children are often easy to spot because they are characteristically pale, thin, below average in growth, and malnour-ished all in the setting of the symptoms described above. Crohn's disease affects 1.4 million Americans, 140,000 under the age of 18. Approximately

---

[55] http://www.naspghan.org/files/documents/pdfs/cme/podcasts/MakingRightIBD Diagnosis.pdf

25% of all new cases in the population are under 20, and roughly 30,000 new patients are diagnosed annually. Remarkably, the incidence is increasing in the Western world especially in children under ten years old.

A study of pediatric patients showed that most were placed on pred-nisone (70%) and mesalamine (61%) in the first month after diagnosis, almost half were placed on immunomodulators, which rose to over 80% by a year. Very young children do not undergo surgery at the same rates as older ones and adults, at least in the United States.[56]

According to the North American Society for Pediatric Gastroenterology, Hepatology and Nutrition, "Monitoring children with UC and CD is not limited to observing symptoms; it also involves assessing weight and height gains, sexual maturation, extra-intestinal manifestations, and psychosocial well-being." It also involves frequent monitoring of blood tests, stool tests and repetition of endoscopy and colonoscopies to assess if treatments are effective.[57]

Treatments include corticosteroids, enteral feeding — liquid diets fed through a tube into the nose — and monoclonal antibodies. They can have serious side effects, especially for child growth and development. [58]

Dr. Dunkin treats patients in an IBD Center at Sinai, created from the formerly separate pediatric and adult divisions, which allows him to continue treating long-time patients instead of handing them off to other specialists. A team approach includes adult and other pediatric GI specialists, nutrition-ists, surgeons, nurses and nurse practitioners, a social worker and two nutri-tionists. The center is also involved in clinical trials. Dunkin is lead investigator at Sinai on a variation of the Viaskin® technology, best known to food allergy patients as the peanut patch, a form of immunotherapy called EPIT — epicutaneous immunotherapy. The hypothesis is that exposing the patient to antigens *via the skin* can lead to the development of protective T regulatory cells (Tregs) that could be migrated to the gut and reduce the destructive immune mechanisms that make Crohn's so miserable.

---

[56] M.E. Schaefer, J.T. Machan, D. Kawatu *et al.*, *"Factors that determine risk* for surgery in pediatric patients with Crohn's disease," *Clinical Gastroenterology* and *Hepatology* 2010; 8(9):789–794, DOI: 10 1016/j cgh 2010 05 021.

[57] http://www.naspghan.org/content/53/en/Inflammatory-Bowel-Disease

[58] http://www.naspghan.org/files/documents/pdfs/cme/podcasts/EN%20Newsltr_WEB.pdf

While both allergies, which react to foreign bodies, and immune-mediated diseases, in which the body may attack its own tissue, are caused by disruption in the normal functioning of innate and acquired immunity, each category is skewed toward one side or the other. Innate immunity, which under ordinary conditions attacks infections from bacteria and viruses, is mediated by Th1 helper cells. Allergies are in effect misplaced actions of acquired immunity, the part that is mobilized by first exposures to infectious diseases and vaccines, mediated by Th2 cells. The T helpers are each responsible for secreting distinctive cytokines that depending on their levels account for particular disorders. If there is too much Th2 activity, allergies are the result. Too much Th1, autoimmunity.

Dr. Dunkin began working with Dr. Li when she noticed that FAHF-2 inhibited production of tumor necrosis factor alpha (TNF-α). High levels of TNF-α were also associated with Crohn's disease. TNF-α increases the transport of white blood cells to inflamed sites where they spur the secretion of tissue-degrading enzymes, causing the damage that can be seen through endoscopy.

High TNF-α levels are found both in the serum and the inflamed mucosa. Serum levels of the cytokine have been shown to align with clinical and laboratory indices of intestinal disease activity. Infliximab, a monoclonal antibody that inhibits secretion of TNF-α, is the first effective biological therapy approved for commercial use. Dr. Dunkin and his co-authors have written that monoclonal antibodies have "revolutionized" treatment of Crohn's. Monoclonal antibodies targeted against IFN-γ (fontolizumab) and IL-17A (secukinumab), two other cytokines that are elevated in Crohn's, were not effective in treating the disease. Infliximab causes adverse reactions in some patients, severe enough to discontinue treatment, although rapid desensitization can restore its safety.[59]

An additional problem with monoclonal antibodies is that they are also very expensive to develop and administer. The most widely used is omalizumab, Xolair, used to treat asthma, chronic urticaria, and as an adjunct to oral immunotherapy for food allergies, at approximately $1,000 per dose. But

---

[59] Ahmad A. Mourad, Moheb N. Boktor, Yesim Yilmaz-Demirdag, Sami L. Bahna, "Adverse reactions to infliximab and the outcome of desensitization," *Annals of Allergy, Asthma, and Immunology August* 2015; 115(2): 87–164.

at least an allergist can give omalizumab in the office setting, although many choose to lay it off on hospitals. For IBD, treatment involves lengthy infusions in hospital facilities at an annual cost of $30–40,000. "What we really need is a pill," Dr. Dunkin says.

Parents think so, too. The IBD center at Sinai surveyed several hundred parents and caregivers about their use of complementary and alternative medical (CAM) treatments. Unlike some such surveys, prayer was omitted from this one because they were interested in possible clashes with the potent treatments administered at the center; prayer has no known contraindications with monoclonal antibodies or steroids.[60]

Thirty-six percent of respondents reported that their children had used CAM, and 19.6% were currently using some form of it. Nearly 40% of respondents had used CAM themselves and 27.7% were currently using it. Almost two thirds were "extremely" or "very supportive" of CAM.

"Unique to this study," the authors say, "was the survey of parents' attitudes to using CAM at the time of their child's diagnosis." Families are supportive of CAM both at the time of initial diagnosis and as an ongoing part of their treatment. They are increasingly aware of side effects from conventional therapy including, "hepatic T-cell lymphoma, increased incidence of skin cancer with thiopurines, and the risk of serious infections with biologic agents."

The first study, which I wrote about in my other book, showed that FAHF-2 has immuno-regulatory effects on human peripheral blood mononuclear cells (PBMCs) and mucosal tissue from Crohn's subjects and in a murine model of colitis, affecting both the adaptive and innate immune systems. FAHF-2 inhibited TNF-α production by PBMCs and mucosa of CD subjects by both monocytes and T cells, suggesting that FAHF-2 targets pathogenic cells secreting inflammatory cytokines. Besides targeting specific pathogenic cells producing TNF-α, FAHF-2 modulates many of the inflammatory cytokines shown to be elevated in CD including IFN-γ, IL-1β, IL-2, IL-6, IL-12 and IL-17.[61]

---

[60] Clare Ceballos, PNP; Ruijun Bao, MD; David Dunkin, MD; Ying Song, MD; Xiu-Min Li, MD; Keith Benkov, MD, "Complementary and alternative medicine use at a single pediatric inflammatory bowel disease center," *Gastroenterology Nursing* 2014; 37(4): 265–271.
[61] Ying Song, MD; David Dunkin, MD; Stephanie Dahan, PhD; Alina Iuga, MD; Clare Ceballos, MS; Kathy Hoffstadter-Thal, MS, MCR; Nan Yang, PhD; Keith Benkov, MD; Lloyd

That suppression of IFN-γ for Crohn's patients is particularly interesting because among food allergy patients, it is too low and needs to be increased, which is exactly what happens when treated with FAHF-2, the same compound.

This indicates that FAHF-2's immuno-modulatory effects vary depending upon the illness. Given the multiple effects, FAHF-2 may indeed be superior to single target medications like monoclonal antibodies and without the side effects seen with corticosteroids and other broad immunosuppressants and monoclonal antibodies.

The anti-inflammatory properties of FAHF-2 may be at least partially attributed to its blocking of the nuclear factor (NF-κB) pathway, which plays a crucial role in pro-inflammatory cytokine production. Inhibiting N-FκB is considered a promising target for intervention in IBD. The mechanism for this was a decrease in IκB-α phosphorylation, i.e., delivery of phosphate to organic compounds. IκB-α phosphorylation and IkB-α degradation might be directly inhibited by FAHF-2 or there may be interference upstream. They concluded that finding the precise means would depend on isolating and studying individual active compounds.

An additional challenge would be to reduce the burden of treatment. FAHF-2's promise as a food allergy treatment was limited by the large number of pills required, sparking the development of a highly refined version — butanol-extracted FAHF-2 or B-FAHF2, described elsewhere in this book.

There was every reason to expect that while their improved day-to-day quality of life would give Crohn's patients plenty of incentive to persist in taking their medicine, too heavy a daily regimen would be a problem. If, as Dr. Dunkin says, we need a pill he acknowledges that there should not be 40 of them if we can help it.

Ganoderic Acid C1 (GAC1)

The most promising herb for inhibiting TNF-α was familiar to Mount Sinai researchers. Ganoderma *lucidum* (G. *lucidum*) is a major constituent both in

Mayer, MD; Xiu-Min Li, MD, MS, "Anti-inflammatory effects of the Chinese herbal formula FAHF-2 in experimental and human IBD," *Inflammatory Bowel Diseases* January 2014; 20(1).

FAHF-2, and anti-asthma herbal medical intervention (ASHMI). Experiments with ASHMI discussed earlier in this book showed it to be as effective as prednisone in treating eosinophilic (allergic) asthma and in a neutrophil-predominant, steroid-resistant asthma model. The therapeutic effect was associated with significant suppression of pro-allergic Th2 cytokines and pro-inflammatory cytokines TNF-α and IL-17.

A number of previous studies reported that polysaccharides from G. *lucidum* modulate cytokines and showed that the triterpenoid fraction of G. *lucidum* was more potent than polysaccharide fractions in suppressing TNF-α. Among 15 isolated triterpenoids, Ganoderic acid C1 (GAC1) was the strongest. A previous experiment had shown that it inhibited TNF-α production by a murine macrophage cell line by down-regulating the NF-κB signaling pathway, which also plays a part in neutrophil-predominant asthma as well as in IBD. They hypothesized that it might also suppress inflammatory responses in IBD, and set out to investigate its potential for suppressing inflammation in Crohn's by inhibiting secretion not just of TNF-α but other pro-inflammatory cytokines from peripheral blood mononuclear cells (PBMCs) and inflamed colonic mucosa from pediatric patients, and by examining how they work.

The experiment took two approaches.

One was to pre-incubate a murine cell line (RAW 254.7) for 24 hours both with GAC1 and without it. This was followed by an additional 24 hours with the Lipopolysaccharide (LPS) from the bacteria *Escherrichia coli*. LPS is found in cell walls and is known to provoke strong immune responses. The ratio of viable cells to total cells was calculated to assure there were no toxic effects of GAC1 on the cells.

The second was done with blood samples taken from 12 pediatric patients diagnosed with Crohn's disease.[62] PBMCs were incubated in culture medium with or without GAC1 for 24 hours. LPS was added and culture conditions maintained for another 24 hours and then supernatants were measured for TNF-α. In parallel experiments that served to look at mechanisms, PBMCs were cultured overnight in serum free medium with or without GAC1. Cells were stimulated with LPS or TNF-α for ten minutes. The ratio of viable cells to total cells was calculated here as well.

---

[62] Study approved by the Institutional Review Board at the Icahn School of Medicine at Mount Sinai. All patients signed informed consent. No patients were on immunomodulating medications including steroids, thiopurines and biologics.

Inflamed colonic biopsies from CD subjects were placed into culture with proportionate volumes of medium based on weight of the specimen with or without GAC1 for 24 hours. Supernatants were filtered and kept for measurement of cytokines.

GAC1 Inhibited TNF-α Production by RAW 264.7 Macrophages

They found that LPS enhanced TNF-α production, and pretreatment with GAC1 decreased it in a dose-dependent manner. GAC1 showed a significant inhibitory effect at concentrations as low as $10\mu g/mL$ and showed no significant cytotoxicity at any dose tested.

GAC1 Suppressed TNF-α Production by PBMCs from CD Subjects

Given the importance that TNF-α plays in the pathogenesis of CD and the inhibitory effects of GAC on TNF-α production *in vitro*, the effect of GAC1 on TNF-α secretion by PBMCs from CD subjects was tested next. LPS significantly enhanced TNF-α production by PBMCs from CD subjects. Simultaneous treatment with GAC1 reduced TNF-α secretion, again, with no cytotoxicity.

GAC1 Suppressed Inflammatory Cytokine Production from Mucosa from CD Subjects

To assess the effects of GAC1 on colonic mucosa, where any medication is likely to have the largest effect, CD-inflamed biopsies and non-CD, normal control biopsies were incubated with and without GAC1 and quantified cytokines levels in the supernatant. Inflamed biopsies from CD subjects had significantly more production of TNF-α and IFN-γ production, compared with non-CD controls. GAC1 significantly suppressed the production of TNF-α, IFN-γ, and IL-17A and showed evidence of inhibiting IL-6 production from the inflamed CD biopsies. CD biopsies showed negligible production of other tested cytokines. GAC1 had no effect on cytokine production from biopsies from control subjects.

GAC1 Inhibited the NF-κB Signaling Pathway in PBMCs

LPS and TNF-α stimulation of cells induces the secretion of pro-inflammatory cytokines through activation of the NF-κB signaling pathway. Phosphorylation of IkB-α was enhanced by both LPS and TNF-α stimulation, but pre-treatment with GAC1 significantly inhibited this phosphorylation.

GAC1 Inhibited the NF-κB Signaling Pathway in the Mucosa

Phosphorylation of IκB-α occurred within ten minutes after cells were stimulated with TNF-α. GAC1 significantly inhibited this phosphorylation. Phosphorylation of IκBα in three inflamed colonic biopsies from CD subjects were also examined by Western blot analysis. Compared with the medium alone group, GAC1 treatment significantly inhibited IκBα activation. These results demonstrate that GAC1 disrupts the NF-κB pathway in PBMCs, colonic biopsies, and lamina propria mononuclear cells, leading to decreased production of TNF-α and other pro-inflammatory cytokines.

These results make GAC1, perhaps in conjunction with other compounds in FAHF-2 and ASHMI, a plausible candidate for study as a Crohn's pill. I asked Dr. Dunkin what is next? More mice? His answer:

> We did a mouse study with FAHF-2. We probably won't do one with GAC1. The next phase is to perform a safety trial in human subjects with Crohn's disease. Once we assure it is safe we will be able to proceed to efficacy trials. It is a long process but one we believe will result in a new, safe treatment option for patients with IBD.

One Mother's Crohn's Story

What is life like for patients with Crohn's and their families? There are no case studies of Crohn's from Dr. Li's practice to draw on, but I reached out to the mother of one patient to find out:

> Outwardly, my son's symptoms presented themselves the very day he turned 6½. However, looking back, I think they started about six months earlier. His kindergarten teacher would joke with me that he never smiled or

laughed at school, a description of which didn't match the silly kid I knew and loved at home. I can't help but wonder if he was hurting inside.

He was tired. Out of the blue, he slept a good portion of every day. He went from being a very active camper at sports camp ("Best Camper" in his age division) to not being able to hold his head up. Nausea and low-grade fevers kicked in. A pattern ultimately developed. He'd be sick for two weeks and close-to-normal for one week before starting the cycle over again. After six weeks, his temperature skyrocketed to 104° or 105°. Our local infectious disease specialist was stumped. He advised taking him to the ER at our local children's hospital right away.

In retrospect, there were other signs.

Unnoticed by us (and apparently his now-former pediatrician), he had fallen off the growth chart for both height and weight. By the time he was hospitalized, he weighed less than 40 lbs. (His then 2½year old brother was quickly catching up [with] him.) He went from outgrowing his shoes every three months or so to wearing the same pair until they wore out. When the GI first told us that my son has moderate to severe Crohn's throughout his entire digestive tract (from esophagus to colon), after the first colonoscopy/endoscopy, I asked him amidst tears if he'll have to give up his plans of becoming a professional hockey player. How could I dash his dreams at such an early age? Without missing a beat, the GI pulled out his cell phone and Googled "NHL players who have Crohn's." They do exist! That's how I knew we found the perfect doctor for us.

So fortunately, his quality of life has not yet been impacted, although steroids have made him puffy. If anything, we spoil him a bit more than we should to somehow make up for mommy and daddy guilt. He's a happy, active and otherwise healthy little boy, who has the world in the palm of his hands. He's currently playing on two hockey teams as the leading goal scorer for both!

This did have an impact on family life.

When he was first diagnosed, I was crushed. My husband was crushed. We had a hard time communicating and needed time to process, independently. But after a few days of paralyzing sadness, I snapped out of it and diverted my anxiety into learning everything there was to know about Crohn's. People came out of the woodwork to tell me about Crohn's in their own families. Knowledge empowered me.

Treatments?

To get symptoms and inflammation under control quickly, he started with a
course of prednisone. The drug selection process is a tough one; there are
no easy answers and they all come with frightening potential side effects.
We went with the immunosuppressant 6MP as his first line of treatment;
however, it quickly caused his liver enzymes to increase. Due to dosing
issues with 6MP, Plan B was a switch to the similar drug of Imuran, plus
allopurinol. If this combo ultimately doesn't pan out, we're likely going to
take a treatment path much less traveled called anti-MAP therapy, which
involves long-term use of antibiotics.

5

MAST CELL ACTIVATION SYNDROME

Mast cells start in the bone marrow as CD34+ progenitor cells — CD34+ being a cell surface marker that identifies this kind of nascent cell. After birth, they are carried by the blood to mucosal tissue that interacts with the environment, the sinuses, lungs, and digestive tract, as well as the skin, where they are the front line of defense against invaders, which is why they figure so heavily in allergies.[63]

They were described in 1878 by Dr. Paul Ehrlich (no relation) who named them under the mistaken belief that they played a role in attracting nutrients to the surrounding tissues the way acorns on the ground or other food sources attract deer during the winter, referred to as the "mast" by hunters. Dr. Thomas Platts-Mills, a major authority on allergies, told me this, along with another bit of lore. Once asked how much space mast cells would occupy if they were collected from all parts of the body, Ehrlich estimated a mass the size of a spleen.[64] According to Platts-Mills, contemporary immunologists still repeat this estimate without its ever having been studied.

---

[63] Joesph Bellanti, MD, *Immunology IV Clinical Applications in Health and Disease* 2012; ICare Press, Bethesda.

[64] How big is a spleen? "An easy way to remember the anatomy of the spleen is the 1×3×5×7×9×11 rule. The spleen is 1" by 3" by 5", weighs approximately 7 oz., and lies between the 9th and 11th ribs on the left hand side." (http://en.wikipedia.org/wiki/Spleen).

As part of innate immunity, mast cells confront infectious agents and ignite a rapid, potent inflammatory response through the release of a soup of mediators. After an initial exposure to an antigen, acquired immunity kicks in. The helper cells create antigen-specific antibodies that recognize particular invaders, allowing the mast cells to react quickly to repeat encounters and eliminate a threat before it spreads. In the case of smallpox, say, or measles, this is a good thing, and is the rationale for vaccination. Unfortunately for allergic people, they can also become sensitized to otherwise harmless antigens such as pollens and certain food proteins.

In addition to allergies, there are other conditions associated with errant mast cells. One is mastocytosis, in which too many mast cells crowd into the available tissue. When activated, they produce symptoms like flushing and intractable urticaria, i.e., hives, in the skin, or worse, depending on where they congregate.[65]

In a 2010 article called "Mast cell activation syndrome: Proposed diagnostic criteria" the authors say that in the late 1980s a new set of disorders were described that were characterized by "sudden synchronous mediator release in the absence of evidence of mast cell proliferation." Twenty-plus years later, voila — those disorders have two names — mast cell activation syndrome (MCAS) or mast cell activation disorder (MCAD).[66]

There is a flood of degranulation in mast cells in different parts of the body producing symptoms involving "the dermis, gastrointestinal tract, and cardiovascular system frequently accompanied by neurologic complaints." Flushing, itching, terrible stomachaches, and spiking blood pressure all at once.

I asked a friend, Tricia Gavankar, a registered nurse who suffers from MCAS, to describe her triggers and symptoms of what she calls "mast cell meltdown."

> Facial products: start[s] with an intense burning sensation. Progress[es] to 'lobster-red facial rash.' Usually followed by abdominal pain or chest tightness.

---

[65] Bellanti, p. 695.

[66] Cem Akin, Peter Valent, Dean D. Metcalfe, "Mast cell activation syndrome: Proposed diagnostic criteria," *Journal of Allergy and Clinical Immunology* 2010; 126(6): 1099–1104.e4.

Food: starts with abdominal pain, facial/mouth/throat/ear itching, abdominal pain, feeling of not being able to swallow.

Pollen/environment: chest tightness, scratchy throat, abdominal pain, facial flushing.

Body lotion: intense burning after taking warm bath. Feels like acid and only solution is to rinse it off immediately. Skin felt prickly, hot.

In general, the few days after an MCAS exposure, flush, event, episode (whatever we call it), I am VERY tired, often have a low blood pressure with dizziness. The elevated histamine levels most likely linger for a few days with MCAS as compared to an IgE reaction.

In a 2011 paper grappling with recognizing the clinical manifestations of MCAS, 18 patients were studied, chosen on the basis of three criteria:

(1) they had at least 4 of 6 clinical features (abdominal pain, diarrhea, flushing, headache, memory and concentration difficulties, and dermatographism), (2) symptoms responded to anti-MC mediator medications, and (3) they had laboratory evidence of MC mediator release.[67]

Sixteen were women between the ages of 20 and 60 at the time of diagnosis and their experience was quite germane for a case treated by Dr. Li starting in 2014. They were symptomatic for about four and a half years during which they were treated by many doctors for many conditions before MCAS was identified.

A review article published in 2013[68] called MCAS a "diagnosis of exclusion" made after ruling out primary and secondary mast cell activation disorders and idiopathic anaphylaxis.

A bone marrow biopsy establishes the diagnosis by revealing the presence of monoclonal mast cells that carry the D816V KIT mutation and/or express

---

[67] Matthew J. Hamilton, Jason L. Hornick, Cem Akin, Mariana C. Castells, Norton J. Greenberger, "Mast cell activation syndrome: A newly recognized disorder with systemic clinical manifestations," *Journal of Allergy and Clinical Immunology* 2012; 128(1): 147–152.e2.

[68] Matthieu Picard, MD; Pedro Giavina-Bianchi, MD, PhD; Veronica Mezzano, MD; Mariana Castells, MD, PhD, "Atopic clinical entities update expanding spectrum of mast cell activation disorders: monoclonal and idiopathic mast cell activation syndromes," *Clinical Therapeutics* 2013; 35(5).

CD25 while the diagnostic requirements for systemic mastocytosis are not met. MCAS affects predominantly women in whom no mast cell abnormality or external triggers account for their episodes of mast cell activation.

"Conventional Treatment" of MCAS

I am using the term "conventional treatment" for MCAS loosely, since the diagnosis itself is essentially brand new and there has not been much time to develop a conventional treatment. The authors of the 2013 article point out that treatment is aimed at "mitigating the effects of mediators released by mast cells on activation and to a certain extent at preventing mediator release" but there is no current curative therapy. Therefore, the goal is to control symptoms and achieve a normal quality of life, based on treatment for systemic mastocytosis starting with histamine-blocking medication, along with medicines that block other mediator release — leukotriene antagonists, cromolyn sodium, and aspirin. A third of treated patients achieved complete resolution, a third had a major response, and a third a minor response. However, no drug trials were done.

Treatment also entails avoiding a menu of prominent triggers including alcohol, heat, drugs such as antibiotics, NSAIDs, narcotics, and neuromuscular blocking agents, radiocontrast media, invasive procedures including general anesthesia, biopsy, endoscopy, hymenoptera stings, fever or infection, exercise, physical stimuli such as pressure, friction, non-steroidal anti-inflammatory drugs, and my favorites "emotions and stress."

Katherine M. — Case Study

Katherine M. glowed when I met her. Nineteen years old, vivacious, confident, and 5'11", there was nothing about her to indicate that six months previously she had been helping her parents plan her own funeral. She and her mother sat across a table in a coffee shop from me where they took turns talking about Katherine's illness, with the occasional admonition from mom for daughter to stop looking at the hot guys who wandered past the window.

Five years earlier, Katherine was a nationally ranked horsewoman in her age bracket for showjumping, and owner of two premier horses. This is an arduous and dangerous sport.

Katherine says that in the fall of 2009 during the State and National Finals season in West Palm Beach, Florida, she began to experience headaches, loss of appetite, and pain during exercise. She was unable to eat without pain and began to vomit.

By the end of November, she returned to her Connecticut home to enroll in school but even without the pressure and physical demands of riding, symptoms persisted.

> Because of my jumping, I didn't do regular sports, but I did work out. In the middle of a workout with the school gym teacher, I vomited, became dizzy, bloated, and was in extreme pain. I didn't know at that point that I had become exercise intolerant. I had to drop out of school shortly after, went to the ER two days later. They found that I was extremely constipated, but had no other help.
>
> From December to May my mother and I went to numerous GI specialists, from Hartford to Boston. I was told that I had IBS, Functional Bowel, or the best one a 'displaced anus.' That's right — they told me that all my symptoms were due to the structure of my bum, which had never been an issue before. What a sad thing to give everything up for! I was discouraged to say the least.

So began a five-year medical odyssey to nowhere. Katherine gave me the three loose-leaf notebooks of paper trail.

This doctor's note is from August 10, 2010:

> Katherine M. presents with complaints of abdominal pain. The patient confirms having constipation, diarrhea and weight loss. The patient denies having chills. Fever, anorexia, hematemesis, melena, bloody stool, dysuria, hematuria, non-menstrual bleeding, pelvic pressure, vaginal discharge, menstrual-type cramping, duration and frequency of periods are abnormal. Patient eats any food and within ten minutes has severe pain in upper outer quadrant of abdomen. She gets severely bloated and is in agony. Has had an upper endoscopy, a CT of the abdomen, has seen a neurologist, a psychologist, and a GI specialist who have not helped her. She has been treated for Lyme disease twice, currently on second course of Doxycycline [antibiotic], and her fatigue has improved, however her abdominal pains continue. Her life, her family's lives have been put on hold due to the severity of her symptoms. She had to drop out of private Prep school in April because her symptoms were so bad. She has been unable to ride. Mom is a

nurse, dad is a dentist and they have done everything in their power to help her. Prior to the start of this she had normal bowel movements. Now they are erratic and she usually has to take a laxative. She is afraid to eat because of the pain. As a last resort she has taken Vicodin very rarely, and this does relieve the pain. She has tried elimination diets, and the GI specialist told her it was all "functional" but did not give her any idea how to help things.

Neurologist found she was positive for cardiolipin AB. Psychologist did not feel she had an eating disorder. She also sees an endocrinologist for thyroid, and is currently on synthyroid 0.5 mg. Parents are at their wits' end.

Laurin, Kate's mother, said later, "I felt helpless. I am a trained nurse. I've been to graduate school. I run a business. Why couldn't I manage to feed my child?" But the search for answers continued. Oddly, it was the family experience with horses that provided the impetus to go on.

We had seen repeatedly that veterinarians would look at symptoms and blame the horse's temperament, or they would want to treat for something that just didn't sound right to us. Eventually we would meet someone who found inflammation in a joint that sounded plausible. We knew our horses and we knew our daughter.

Over the next several months, Kate was given genetic tests; tests for epidermal nerve fiber density (a clinical note said the lab did not have normal values for the patient's age); she tested Negative for G20210A [2nd most common risk factor for thrombosis]; "Heterogeneous for A1298C, and neg. for C677T" and for Antiphospholipid Antibody Syndrome.

In September, 2010 Katherine saw a neurologist who reported:

17-year-old female patient with abdominal pain diffuse for 1 day. The symptoms are severe, additional symptoms or pertinent history also N.V.; headache. Furthermore, the patient/family denies anorexia; fever; genital pain, back pain; dysuria, cough, sob. She has had 2 years of bad pain, worse after eating. She was diagnosed with celiac artery compression, and ischematic duodenum. She had surgery to fix it but still has pain. She has been diagnosed with gastroparesis and a leaky gut and has multiple food allergies and only eats vegetables and fish. She gets dehydrated easily and improves with rehydration.

In a letter to the primary care physician, this specialist noted:

> Neurological examination showed slender physique, mild disturbance of memory and confusion evident in conversation, tightness of cervical paraspinal muscles, slight scoliotic curvature, tremor of the hands in sustension, hypoactive arm and knee reflexes, Romberg sign, and tandem imbalance with intact cranial nerves and absent Babinski signs.

It continued:

> The findings were consistent with dysautonomia manifesting OTS, sudomotor dysautonomia and gastrointestinal complaints; in association with headache, cognitive, and emotional complaints indicating CMS involvement; thyroid endocrinopathy, prior recent head trauma; analgesic tolerance for pain; and presumed Lyme exposure.

Katharine's own timeline of her illness, sent to me via email, is as follows:

November 9th 2010 — Hartford Hospital Celiac Mesenteric Artery Study
"Velocity decrease with inspiration is suggestive of median arcuate ligament compression"

November 12th 2010 — General doctor wants to do a GI with small bowel Follow through
Test shows delayed gastric emptying
Abnormally dilated duodenum with dysfunctional peristalsis

November 30th — Because of suggestion of MALS and severity of vomiting and pain, went to NYU. Saw Dr. XXXX
Ordered further testing

December 6th — MRI Angiogram with contrast
Positive for Median Arcuate Ligament Compression Syndrome

December 12th — Went to meet Dr. So-and-So at NYU (specializes in gastric bypass) one of the very few that can perform the surgery
Made surgery arrangements.

December 24th — Had a successful surgery

December 27th–Jan 2nd — Withdrew off my normal 7, 7.5 Vicodin a day cold turkey. Wanted. To. Die.

Jan 2nd — Left for Florida[,] spent about three months. I did not experience the intolerable pain that I felt with the compression. But, eating food was still extremely uncomfortable for me and I vomited often due to fear of feeling terrible and bloating

April 18th — Headed home from Florida in hopes that I could learn how to eat normally and heal

Still experiencing pain and nausea with eating[,] general doctor checks for gallbladder

Inconclusive

The focus now became my weight seeing as I weighed in at about 113 and was 5'11. How to get food into me became my main priority

June 9th 2011 — Went to a ND Dietician who did an IgG allergy test

Sensitive to 72 foods, recommended I do not eat any of them

End of June 2011 — began taking IVIG (intravenous gamma globulin) prescribed by neurologist to heal my "small nerve damage" in hopes that it would also help the small intestine work better

*Began riding again

Fall 2011 continued with restricted diet of fish, shrimp and lettuce and treatment of IVIG

Went back to college

Decided to see Dr. ****** to help me with nutrition and supplements

Decided to test me for parasites

Went for a colon scrape

Colon was red inflamed with large amounts of Charcoal Leyden Crystals, although the exact amoeba was not found there was enough evidence to treat for parasites

Jan 2012 — Dr. ******* encouraged me to expand my diet, due to heavy metal poisoning from my restricted diet.

Tried to expand my diet for two months, my symptoms were so severe that I unintentionally lost weight to the point of 98 lbs.

March 19th 2012 — Decided to go to inpatient treatment at (residential center for girls with eating disorders)

Gained 25 lbs 5 weeks[69]

From May to fall of 2012 I struggled with having terrible intolerances to food. My bloating was terrible, broke out with rashes and cystic acne, and vomited for relief of how terrible I felt almost every day.

Fall 2012–Spring 2013

Fall — I struggled a lot but made it through school.

Spring — I took 4 classes and realized that if I lived on adrenaline rather than vomit I could stop vomiting. For three months I didn't vomit, barely slept, but felt a relief of my symptoms. One day during a reaction I decided to try Benadryl. I felt so much better, by the summer I was living on 12 Benadryl a day.

Fall 2013 — I began to crash it seemed that I couldn't keep myself on an adrenaline high forever. I was going to the hospital at least once a week to get rehydrated and the only food I was able to eat without vomiting was duck eggs. My mother and I went to the GI group at Yale that were so concerned with my symptoms that they recommended that I go to the Mayo Clinic for further diagnostics. We called but the wait was at least three months. My mother found a specialist GI doctor in (another city). We went straight to the ER I was hospitalized with a potassium of 2.7 with heart complications.

I stayed in the hospital for four days. I did not eat. It baffled everyone how much better I did if I didn't have food. No food, no reactions. On the fourth day, Dr. B***** gave me a consultation and told us to consider something bigger than just what could be happening with my digestion.

My mom looked up possibilities and stumbled upon mastocytosis, the symptoms were so similar to what I experienced.

Mother and daughter packed the car and hit the road. "I told my husband, we're not coming back till we have a diagnosis," her mom told me. The trip was frustrating. They drove to Pittsburgh where a mastocytosis specialist told Katie with his best bedside manner, "If you don't get better you'll never

---

[69] This was a particularly grim episode. By Kate's account, some of the other girls were quite disturbed. They would pull out various tubes that had been inserted to keep them alive and prowl around in the night like Dracula's women. Her mother told me, "She said, forcing myself to eat just to gain weight there was like trying to have sex after being raped."

qualify for life insurance." They drove straight through from Pittsburgh to Boston overnight, stopping only at every bathroom they could find along the way. Mom was stopped for speeding but a sympathetic trooper let them go when he saw Kate with a bucket of vomit in her lap.

Boston seemed like a great option because they have the Center for Mastocytoscis at Brigham and Woman's. But they wanted a positive tryptase test to be seen by their doctors. Not possible on short notice.

Discouraged, they went home. Kate says,

My sister and her fiancé drove from college to be with me, I didn't see the point in living anymore. I suggested that I take five days off from eating, and because my symptoms were so bad my whole family supported it. With nowhere else to turn, my mom emailed Dr. M******** at Mount Sinai who immediately called her back and told her to bring me in, and that he would do the blood tests. He said I didn't seem like a classic mastocytocis patient and referred me to Dr. Mirna Chehade at Mount Sinai in New York. Dr. Chehade was great. I told her my situation and that sometimes I just don't want to keep going. I will never forget her response[,] she said, with a smile, "If you ever feel like that you call me. You can't die because of a bad stomach, you have to pick a way more glamorous reason to die!" Dr. Chehade scoped me and put me on a hypoallergenic baby shake (which I threw up every time). She called and said that she knew the doctor for me.

Winter 2013 — Enter Dr. Anne Maitland.

Anne Maitland is both an MD and a PhD. She claims that key to her interest in diagnosing and treating patients with mast cell activation disorders lies in the difference between the ways she was trained to think for the two degrees. She says, "MDs are taught to profile patients. PhDs are taught to ask the right questions." Instead of treating, say, atopic dermatitis or asthma as they become symptomatic, she learned to investigate the ties between these conditions. "The immune system, the respiratory system, and the digestive system are all tied together by the nervous system."

Anne is a close reader of Dr. Jerome Groopman, who writes about medicine for *The New Yorker*. She was heavily influenced by his 2000 article "Hurting All Over" about fibromyalgia, which I read after talking to her. It introduced me to the term "wastebasket disease" — so-called because it was defined out of a complex of complaints that could not be attributed to any established diseases diagnosable or treatable by specialists. That certainly comports with the maze of physical and mental blind alleys that Kate had encountered over five years.

One passage of Groopman's 2000 article particularly describes Maitland's approach:

> Language is as vital to the physician's art as the stethoscope or scalpel. A doctor begins by examining the words of his patient to determine their clinical significance. He then translates the words into medical language, describing how the condition came to be, what it means, and how it may evolve. Of all the words a doctor uses, the name he gives the illness has the greatest weight. It forms the foundation of all subsequent discussion, not only between doctor and patient but also between doctor and doctor and between patient and patient.

In Dr. Maitland's view, echoing what Groopman says, there's a feeling that "if you can't test for something, it doesn't exist." The time pressures of doctor-patient interaction compound the dilemma. Among many other attributes, Dr. Maitland is a great listener. Like another allergist whom I have interviewed, Dr. Renata Engler, Maitland believes that somewhere along the line, many doctors have come to neglect patient stories. Maitland says, "This has created a desert in which snake oil finds a niche." She can be fierce with the snake-oil crowd, challenging sales reps flogging herbal products over the counter in health food stores to present evidence of the benefits they are promoting. By 2013, Maitland had begun to develop a reputation for diagnosing and treating mast cell disorders, after seeing a number of patients with connective tissue disease, but for whom data did not support a diagnosis of typical food allergies or of mastocytosis. In these patients, the skin, the gut, and the lungs, where the body confronts the environment, were all reactive.

Her fellow allergists, she believes, miss this diagnosis because they are primarily focused on the adaptive or acquired immune system. They test for IgE-mediated mast cell disorders, which are responsible for most atopy, and neglect the larger functioning of the mast cell in innate immunity. She says, "the immune system is like the Bible. It has an Old Testament and a New

Testament. Studying only IgE-mediated mast cell activation is like studying the Bible only through the lens of the New Testament."

Shifting metaphors, Anne says that mast cells do not start life as a problem. Trained as first responders at our borders to the outside world,

> mast cells go through basic training, then are shipped out and stationed to different parts of our bodies. So rookie mast cells stationed in the skin differentiate to the needs of that skin environment, compared to mast cells situated in the gut or respiratory tract. Similar to a new recruit sent to a base in Hawaii versus Iraq.

Mast cells can become dangerous if a subset of them "goes rogue or mast cells are being great soldiers, but following bad orders." Armies of rogue mast cells are rare (mastocytosis), but most allergists are familiar with mast cells following bad orders, such as reacting to IgE targeting harmless substances or allergens.

> Patients with connective tissue disorders appear to have mast cells that are following bad orders, but we just haven't figured out where these bad orders are coming from — the surrounding connective tissue, the local nerves, other local components of the immune system.

When Kate arrived, 5'11" and under 100 pounds, bearing the hundreds of pages of clinical notes and test results that are excerpted above, and the bleakest prognosis imaginable, Maitland thought about something she had learned in a rotation at Rhode Island Children's Hospital: "Try not to steal patients' hope." She asked Kate to talk about her history of symptoms, tests, and treatment in her own words. She heard the story with alternating sympathy and outrage, particularly Kate's account of her month in the residential eating disorder clinic eating junk food, surrounded by desperate girls. Laurin says, "The first thing Dr. Maitland did was to apologize for all the missed diagnoses."

Unnamed Malady

According to Kate,

> Dr. Maitland listened to me, did an examination, and was so strongly convinced about my Mast Cell Activation Disorder that she put me on meds

and also a hypoallergenic diet. My symptoms didn't get better, but they stopped worsening so that alone was encouraging. My next appointment she said, "I think you need to meet Dr. Li, maybe she can help you."

As is the case with some of the patients Groopman has written about over the years, Maitland finds that treatment begins when the doctor says to the patient, "I believe you." For five years, Kate had symptoms without a real name, although it had many aliases. The key to the diagnosis of MCAS was the favorable response to Benadryl. Maitland says, "She took that on her own. No doctor suggested it. It was just something she saw on a shelf at 7-11. To me this was a sure indicator of mast cell involvement." But the effects of Benadryl, an antihistamine, are very temporary and they diminish with constant use.

Maitland spent part of her fellowship in the laboratory of Dr. Xiu-Min Li at Mount Sinai where she was impressed with the quality of the data. She was also impressed with Dr. Li's emphasis on the simultaneous working of multiple body systems rather than their separate functions and malfunctions. She felt that various medicines could be employed to quiet what she calls "anger" in different parts of the body — connective tissue inflammation, GI distress, skin problems, and bronchoconstriction, for example, all tied together by the nervous system through red-alert stress levels — but that addressing them simultaneously would be preferable. She told Kate, "I can treat you, but I know someone who might be able to cure you."

Maitland was so impressed with Dr. Li's treatment that she had opened her suburban office for the latter's use on weekends, and begun to study acupuncture and acupressure, particularly for their use in relieving patient stress. She says, "Those acupuncture and acupressure points are located close to concentrations of mast cells."

Kate looked forward to her first meeting with a degree of skepticism, bred by years of experience, "As you know from reviewing my case, I have seen a lot of different specialists, and even a couple different acupuncturists, so I wasn't skeptical of her treatment, I think I just didn't believe any plan would work for me." That began to change when they met. "I must say when I first looked at her, she had wisdom that seemed to exude out of her, the kind of smarts you can feel without first reviewing her credentials."

For her part Dr. Li's first impression was that Kate looked "terrible." This was pretty strong language for this particular doctor in my experience and it certainly did not correspond to the vivacious young woman I met six months later. What did "terrible" mean? It meant she was in pain, feeling hopeless, too weak to stand up for very long. She was bloated from malnourishment.

"I had never seen 'MCAS'" Xiu-Min says, "but I had seen all her symptoms, except she claimed she couldn't eat anything but apples." Kate had one in her purse and Dr. Li asked her to eat it. Says Kate, "Dr. Li watched. My, face and hands went red, my feet turned blue, my veins developed a lacey pattern, my stomach bloated, I was in pain, and became dizzy and out of it."

Dr. Li says, "When the apple turned her leg purple…that was new to me."

In light of the importance Dr. Maitland placed on giving MCAS a name, and her confidence that Dr. Li would be able to help, it made sense for me to ask Dr. Li if MCAS has a TCM name.

> No…But the symptoms have names. Fatigue, which everyone with mast cell activation disorders seems to have. Rash. GI problems. You do not need a name to treat these things. Western medicine is very good for diagnosis and understanding how diseases work. TCM is a system of tools and methods to deal with the human condition. This is important because some MCAS symptoms seem to be triggered by everything. Latex is a big one but some people have no IgE to it. That doesn't mean the reaction is all in the patient's head.
>
> I don't look at the clinical record. I look at 'my information.' I look at their skin and their eyes. I listen to their complaints. Patients do a good job of giving you the big picture when you ask, 'What can I do for you? How can I help you?' Looking at clinical notes locks you into what other doctors have already seen.

Kate said that she was unable to do any normal activities. She could not visualize her "real" life and could only focus on current problems. She had not been to school for a long time.

The worst was vomiting. As Dr. Li says:

> She couldn't process proteins in meat at all. She couldn't take a shower because she couldn't tolerate heat. It made her so tired she had to sit down.

She couldn't exercise. TCM helps you recognize syndromes — combinations of symptoms that are associated with different organ systems. They can be treated with different herbs. But we don't necessarily give names to these things.

As Kate's mother remembers it, Dr. Li said, "There are many things wrong. It will take at least a year to fix them. You will continue to take your other medications — they can work together with TCM. We have to start. What is one thing you would like me to do today?"

Dr. Li says,

> I wanted her to feel good. She felt so unhappy, so frustrated, so hopeless. I have confidence in my work and I wanted her to feel like she was in good hands. This is important for all my work because I am asking patients to do things that are very different for them. So I gave her acupuncture.

Laurin says, "Dr. Li said to Kate, 'you lie down' and to me she said, 'you go take a nap.' When I came back, Katie was crying. The acupuncture hurt but it felt like progress."

Dr. Li says, "Then we set the digestion as first goal. We wanted her to stop losing food, stop her vomiting. There would be no medications for the mast cells until she felt better."

Recognizing that Kate has a hard-charging temperament, Dr. Li cautioned her, "Try to save 40% of your energy every day. Don't wear yourself out. When you think about doing the next thing, try to hold back. Don't NOT do it, but don't try so hard."

Still, with all the years of misery, compliance was not a given. I can understand this. TCM is so alien that even a severely ill patient may resist the behavioral changes that treatment requires.

As Kate wrote,

> After my first appointment, I still didn't trust her, or her herbs, but I did open my mind to the idea that maybe she could help. Even though it seems miniscule, as a person with chronic undiagnosable issues, opening your mind to help is a hard step. The fear of being let down again is somewhat crippling, for me it was because I wasn't sure how many more times I could be let down before the thought in my mind of giving up, of killing myself

actually would become actions. As I write this now, it seems somewhat melodramatic but in that period, there was little left of life that didn't cause me pain. I not only couldn't do what I loved anymore, I was beginning to forget the things I loved. Dr. Li sent me off the first day after seeing her with one bottle of digestive tea and bath additives.

When Kate returned for follow up, Dr. Li instantly saw that she had not been taking her medicines. "If you can't see results," she says, "your method is wrong or people aren't taking their medication. I knew the meds would stop vomiting and if she was still vomiting she wasn't taking it. That had to start before we could work on the cells."

Kate's mother recalls Dr. Li saying,

You vomited not once but many times — you couldn't be taking the meds. But you are too sick not to give it a try. You have nothing to lose but you can get your life back. You don't have to be perfect. You, your mother, and I are a team.

Kate later also confessed that she avoided her baths because she associated them with painful heat-triggered episodes.

Dr. Li told me passionately that if I was to see results from her herbs I had to completely follow the protocol and not just every now and again pop a couple teas when I mustered up the courage. That appointment was also pivotal because as I laid on the acupuncture bed she told me to close my eye and imagine myself better, I cried because I truly couldn't after all the years couldn't imagine a better me. But after her talk I adhered to her plan completely and quickly saw results.

She now recalls:

After Dr. Li's strong urging to take my pills and lotions as directed, I followed this plan. Five pills of digestive tea, 3 pills of good mood tea, 1–2 baths a day, and lotion applied to my body morning and night. I did this and ate organic and extremely healthy with no restrictions and a lot of rest. Most of what I was eating was vegan just because I didn't want to challenge my system with the usual allergy offenders. The first week I began to feel much, much better. It is hard to describe the out-of-control and restless feeling you get when you are experiencing 5–6 reactions a day. By the end of the first week my reactions had stopped I went from sleeping 2–3 hours a night to sleeping 8–12. My focus changed and I became relaxed. The pain with eating began subsiding the second week and I experienced a confidence with food I hadn't felt for years. With MCAS food easily becomes your enemy and you could say the animosity between myself and food ran deep. With Dr. Li's pills and no reactions I began enjoying my meals and actually began feeling energy for the first time in years. The biggest thing for me was the difference in vomiting, before Dr. Li I would vomit up to 17 times a day. It took a huge toll on my quality of life and made having energy nothing more than a wish. I reported back to Dr. Li the next month that I hadn't vomited and had no reactions. It was amazing, truly a miracle. My body seemed to not only absorb and use Dr. Li's meds, but have a desperation for them. I think of myself before Dr. Li in a desert of pain and reactions with no water, and Dr. Li's plan to be my oasis, a place of rest and hydration. Speaking of hydration, during the first month I drank 7 liters of water a day I don't know if it is significant for MCAS but for me it was amazing. My friends and family were overjoyed for me and for the first time in years at peace. When the people that love you watch you unable to eat and drown in your own pain[,] every day is a crisis.

Dr. Li says that as bad as Katie's case was,

I have seen worse cases. People who can't walk or talk when they are having an attack. None of their symptoms respond to steroids. You have a new strategy every month or week. Some vomit some don't. Sore throats. Their muscles ache. One woman said she felt like someone had been beating her and her muscles looked like it. They react to chemicals. One lady had a facial and her whole world turned upside down.

Katie and I were both very lucky. I was able to treat her with medications for digestion, and food allergies. These other cases will take additional strategies.

Chapter

6

OBESITY

In her introduction for this book, Dr. Li mentions that the challenge to medicine and to TCM in this post-dynastic era is the proliferation of "good life" diseases. While most of Dr. Li's research concerns maladaptive immunity, the most visible good life disease is obesity, which has more than doubled worldwide over the past couple of decades. To appreciate the spread of this epidemic, you can look at China itself, where obesity has been diagnosed at 25% of the adult population and rising, although still well below US levels. Most of this rise is among the affluent, whose consumption of meat approaches 30% of their diet, five times 1960s levels.[70]

Symptoms cannot be hidden with makeup or treated in the short term. The standard treatments are diet, exercise and behavior modification. Most adults in the United States are either trying to lose weight or to maintain their weight, but few of them have the discipline to make a sustainable dent.

Looking back at the long history of TCM and its contribution to contemporary health, weight loss may not have the cachet of, say, treating wounds and burns in the pharmacopeia that has inspired treatments for eczema, but you only have to look at art from some of the old dynasties to

---

[70] http://blogs.wsj.com/chinarealtime/2011/07/18/study-china-getting-fatter-but-not-like-u-s/?mod=WSJBlog&mod=chinablog

know that obesity is not entirely a modern phenomenon. Some depictions of Confucius show a man who could have stood to lose a few pounds.

The *New York Times* reported in 2015 that because insurers are now covering obesity treatment, consultants have sprung up to teach primary-care doctors how to bill for it, at $3,000 per patient. Major medical centers complain that diet clinics often employ tactics like vitamin injections, supplements and extreme diet plans that sell well but yield no lasting results.[71]

With obesity growing as a threat to public health, there is growing interest in TCM's reputation for safety, efficacy and low cost for weight loss. However, experimental evidence-based studies of oral TCM formulations have been limited and underlying mechanisms are lacking. *Ma Huang* — ephedra — was a staple of many diet aids, but it is no longer sold as it has been shown to pose significant central nervous system and cardiovascular risks. Ephedra-derived weight-loss medicines made headlines in the winter of 2003 because they were linked to the death of a minor league baseball pitcher at spring training with the Baltimore Orioles, as well as previous fatalities in other sports. The *Kampo* formulations used for centuries by Japanese practitioners can result in fatal liver or kidney failure, and pneumonia and pneumonitis have been reported with the use of *Saiboku-to*.

Building on their understanding of metabolic mechanisms and principles of TCM formulation, Dr. Li and her team developed weight-loss herbal intervention therapy (W-LHIT), also known as WL-1, which they tested on mice using rodent models of obesity induced by high-fat-diet (HFD), which have provided a window into disease pathogenesis and useful preclinical models for investigation. W-LHIT consists of 6 Chinese herbal medicines, *Ganoderma lucidum (Ling Zhi), rhizome of Coptis chinensis (Huang Lian), Radix astragali (Huang Qi), Nelumbo nucifera Gaertn (He Ye), Chaenomeles speciosa (Mu Gua), Fructus Aurantii (Zhi Qiao)*. Several have been reported to have anti-obesity effects in animal models, while others reduced the serum glucose level in diabetic mice, and one, *Chaenomeles sinensis*, also showed the ability to lower cholesterol and blood sugar.[72]

---

[71] R. Abrams, K. Thomas, "In Health Law, a Boon for Diet Clinics," *NY Times* July 4, 2015, A-1.

[72] Nan Yang, Danna Chung, Changda Liu, Banghao Liang, Xiu-Min Li, "Weight loss herbal intervention therapy (W-LHIT) a non-appetite suppressing natural product controls weight and lowers cholesterol and glucose levels in a murine model," BMC *Complementary and Alternative Medicine* 2014; 14: 261.

While all have been investigated individually in obesity-related research, they failed to be effective for significant weight loss in short periods of treatment. The objective of this study was to investigate the combined formula on body weight, food consumption, and the weight of epididymal fat tissue — fat that lines part of the male reproductive anatomy that can be harvested and measured as a unit. In addition, they observed the effect on serum glucose, cholesterol, and the expression of two genes, PPARγ and FABP4, involved in metabolic pathways.

The test used fourteen-week-old high-fat-diet induced obese and normal chow fed C57BL/6 J mice. Dried aqueous extracts of the six Chinese herbal medicines were herbs were extracted with water and then concentrated and dried according to the standard decocting and drying manufacturing process. Each mouse received 84 mg W-LHIT daily, dissolved in 1 mL drinking water, and intragastrically (i.g.) administered two separate feedings four hours apart using a standard mouse feeding needle. The W-LHIT dose was determined by a conversion table of equivalent human to animal dose.

They used two protocols in two sets of experiments for weight control.

Experiment 1

The first set was designed to determine the effect of W-LHIT on weight loss as added-on therapy to dietary calorie reduction. Three groups of age matched 14 week-old mice (equivalent to human age of 19 years) were first sham treated with water while continuing on the high-fat diet for three weeks. This acclimatized mice to i.g. administration. Sham-treated normal weight mice were fed a normal fat diet served as controls. Three weeks later, all mice were weighed. Group 1 obese mice continued on HFD and sham treatment as the obesity control group (OB/HFD/Sham). Both group 2 and 3 obese mice were switched from HFD to NFD, but group 2 mice received W-LHIT (OB/NFD/W-LHIT) whereas group 3 mice received water sham treatment (OB/NFD/Sham). Group 4, the normal weight mice, continued on NFD and water sham treatment to serve as normal controls (Normal/NFD/Sham). Treatment duration was ten days. Body weight and food consumption amounts were recorded three times a week. Weight gain was calculated by subtracting body weight on the first day from that on the last day of treatment. Daily body weight gain was calculated by dividing body weight gain by the number of treatment days. Chow was weighed three times a week during the period of acclimatization and treatment, and daily food consumption was calculated by dividing total food consumption by the number of days. Since this was a preliminary study designed to determine whether W-LHIT as add-on therapy enhances normal diet intervention weight loss in young obese mice, they did no biochemistry analysis for serum cholesterol and glucose levels in Experiment 1.

Experiment 2

This one employed older animals. Fourteen-week-old mice were maintained for nine weeks on HFD until 23 weeks old (roughly equivalent to 40 human years). Like the younger set, they were then fed water intragastrically for two weeks. These 25 week-old obese mice were divided into 2 weight-matched groups. Group 1 mice continued on HFD and sham treatment as obese controls (OB/HFD/Sham) while group 2 mice continued on HFD and received W-LHIT treatment (OB/HFD/W-LHIT). Treatment duration was 30 days. Normal weight mice fed with NFD and water sham treatment were used as normal controls (Normal/NFD/Sham). In Experiment 2, mice were starved overnight after 30 days of treatment and submandibular blood samples were collected. Sera were separated and stored at −80°C for further analysis. The mice were sacrificed and tissues were harvested, weighed, and stored at −80°C for further analysis. Serum cholesterol and glucose levels were measured. Epididymal fat pads were collected and weighed. Total RNA was extracted from epididymal fat tissue using Trizol reagent.

Acute toxicity was tested by feeding naïve mice with ten times the daily therapeutic dose for mice of W-LHIT and observed for 14 days. For sub-chronic toxicity, naïve mice were fed five times their daily therapeutic dose for 14 days. Their blood was tested and organs preserved for analysis.

Results

In the first experiment, mice lost body weight when switched from a high-fat diet to a normal-fat diet. W-LHIT formula treatment accelerated daily weight loss by 250%. This finding suggests that, if the same occurred in humans, W-LHIT as part of a dietary weight loss regimen might help young obese patients lose weight more quickly.

In the second experiment, they found that W-LHIT suppressed daily body weight gain in older mice by approximately 800% compared to sham treatment. W-LHIT consistently reduced epididymal fat weight. If W-LHIT were to have the same effects in humans, W-LHIT might help limit weight gain without appetite suppressants and diets. Sounds like a win-win to me. An additional significant outcome in middle-aged mice was reduction of blood cholesterol and glucose levels. If the same results occur in humans, W-LHIT may be valuable in treating pre-metabolic syndrome and perhaps metabolic syndrome.

The researchers suggest a number of explanations for these exciting results. Since W-LHIT reduced body weight gain and normalized cholesterol and glucose levels without suppressing appetite in the middle-aged mice that were eating lots of fat, they hypothesized that it may affect signaling pathways involved in cholesterol and glucose metabolism.

Fatty-acid-binding protein (FABP4) is predominantly expressed in adipose tissue. Recent research found that adipose tissue in obese individuals exhibited lower FABP4 gene expression than adipose tissue from lean individuals. We found that adipose tissue FABP4 gene expression was significantly increased by W-LHIT treatment. This increased FABP4 expression might have led to the decreased glucose levels and body weight.

The treatment showed increased expression of genes tied to mitochondrial fatty acid oxidation (CPT1, UCP2) energy metabolism (AMPK).

Previous research showed that activation of PPARγ is mainly involved in regulating lipid metabolism, insulin sensitivity, and glucose homeostasis and its agonist has been used in the treatment of hyperlipidemia and type 2 diabetes. PPARγ reduces cholesterol synthesis and is also important in energy metabolism.

These genes also play a part in insulin sensitivity and fat formation.

The benefits to human health and vanity from a safe, herbal drug that would make it easy to control weight are so obvious that they take no study or special knowledge to appreciate. Before you start dreaming about losing weight while sticking to a Häagen-Dazs diet, however, one of the researchers on this paper, Dr. Danna Chung, cautioned that the human equivalent of the mouse dosage would be 50 pills twice a day. This is a work in progress.

FUTURE RESEARCH

Dr. Xiu-Min Li

Our research agenda is a combination of past, present and future. I have said that our clinical practice informs our research, which in turn influences the clinical practice. I will now describe how this works.

One part is Clinical Observational Study. That is, research that can be done in concert with the work of our clinic. As I discussed in my introduction, we function under a dual regulatory system, which allows us to use versions of medicines that are not yet approved as pharmaceutical drugs in the form of supplements. It is part of my personal mission to operate on both tracks because the suffering I see in my clinic is so severe. Parents are so anxious to relieve their children's misery that they are taking a chance on our work. I do not feel right about telling all these eczematous, asthmatic, food-allergic children to wait.

Regarding classic clinical trials, not only are blinded placebo-controlled trials very expensive, for some medications they do not make any sense at least until there is proof of concept that would justify a bigger study.

Project 1

The first of these is the bio-marker study discussed briefly in the chapter "Food Allergy Update". One set of patients who will be studied have multiple food allergy sensitizations and history of severe food allergy reactions, they have been practicing avoidance of offending foods, and have infrequent accidental exposure-induced reactions. Despite avoidance, their IgE levels (sensitization) remain very high — above 17.6 KU/L. In some cases, their IgE levels even continue to increase.

A second set are those who have a history of severe reactions and elevated specific IgE levels or whose skin tests are strongly positive. Despite strict avoidance, these food-allergic children experience frequent and potentially severe food-induced anaphylaxis (>10 reactions and >2 epinephrine uses in the three months prior to starting TCM therapy). Attempts to avoid ingestion of offending foods are not sufficient in these patients because their anaphylaxis can also be triggered by inhalation and skin exposure.

In both population groups, the likelihood of naturally outgrowing their food allergy is low.

Although oral food challenge is the gold standard procedure for diagnosis of food allergy, patients with a history of severe reactions are reluctant to undergo baseline food challenge because of the concern of severe reactions. Thus, in this study there will be no challenge at baseline. Biomarkers will provide a powerful tool to predict allergic status at baseline.

The published retrospective case study of three patients (also mentioned in the first chapter) reported that TCM therapy effectively prevented frequent and severe reactions and reduced IgE levels. Further anecdotal data indicates that TCM can reverse the trend of continuing elevation of IgE levels in such patients, and even reduce them. However, it is not possible to predict if an individual will or not react to food that caused previous reactions on the basis of IgE data or even a positive skin test. Biomarkers will provide a powerful tool to assess progress by identifying the relationship between treatment methods and efficacy. If patients' immunological responses are dramatically improved compared to baseline, and if the family is interested in introducing certain foods, allergists will determine clinical tolerability by oral challenge, the clinical practice standard, for assessing food allergy outgrowth.

In this study, TCM treatment will use further refined B-FAHF-2, consisting of concentrated effective fractions of B-FAHF-2 as a dietary supplement. The dose will be twice daily doses of three pills for ages 6–12 and above, two pills for ages 3–5 years and one pill for three year olds and under. The new protocol will be using a two-phase therapy. The first will focus for six months on silencing effector cells such as IgE-bound basophils and mast cells. The goal is to increase clinical tolerance and reduce the risk of reactions following accidental exposure (for example, reducing the frequency and severity of random hives/rash). No challenges will be performed in this stage.

The second phase will focus on immunomodulation of memory T cells and B cells (IgE producing cells) to switch them from allergic to tolerogenic status (long-term effect) and will require two years, which further reduces effector cell activation. Full treatment takes two and a half years, three months shorter than our previous protocol.

This will be a real-world study. In the real world, patients with such severe food allergies in both sub-groups are likely to also have co-existing conditions such as eczema, asthma, allergic rhinitis, or indigestion (stomach pain, abnormal bowel movements). The proposal will allow using additional treatment regimens for these conditions, regimens that have not been notably successful in moderating anaphylaxis in the past. The B-FAHF-2 will be the constant.

Although each sub-project will only include a small number of patients (ten treated patients plus ten control samples of blood) to start with, it can be easily expanded because in this type of clinical-based study, we can just add new patients who fit the profile as new subjects.

Project 2

Practice-based study of traditional Chinese medicine (Chinese herbal medicine and acupuncture/acupressure) effects on steroid-dependent eczema. This is to build on the work described in an earlier chapter.

The overall goal of this study is to use existing traditional Chinese medicine treatments including Chinese herbal medicines, acupuncture/acupressure to improve asthma and eczema control and reduce or eliminate corticosteroid use, and improve overall immune health. Patients 3–12 years old who have been using topical steroids for more than three months and/ or systemic steroids eight days per month, with a history of relapse after cutting back, with total IgE above 1,000 K/L and peanut or other food-specific IgE above 15 K/L. Based on our clinical observations, we expect TCM will improve eczematous lesions and itching by 50–100% within three months and that these gains will persist for the full 12 months of study. Another study is planned to focus on infant and young children ages six months to three years who have eczema and multiple food allergen sensitization, and have used topical steroids for more than three months. Younger children respond to the combined TCM treatment sooner.

Project 3

Practice-based study of Chinese herbal formulas for alleviation of adverse gastrointestinal effects of food allergy and food oral immunotherapy (OIT).

The background for this study is that oral immunotherapy for food allergies — introducing minute quantities of a food allergen into the diet and gradually increasing them to a desired level of unresponsiveness — has become fairly common both in research and in a number of private allergy practices around the country. Unfortunately, this results in a statistically significant number of patients suffering adverse reactions, sometimes severe enough to discontinue treatment. My practice now has seen ample numbers of these patients from both research trials and from practice, some of whom continue their treatment and some who have quit but whose symptoms persist.

While OIT is still not an approved therapy for general allergy practice, and may only ever be offered in specialty practices by doctors who are prepared for round-the-clock coverage of patients who are dosing themselves at home, it has gained momentum and is likely to be one of the choices patients will have available in years to come. Since we can already see the weaknesses of immunotherapy as well as the strengths, exploring the adjunctive, supportive possibilities for TCM as well as the remedial ones makes sense.

Project 4

Practice-based study to develop biomarkers to complement current lab tests in an attempt to enhance the ability to diagnose allergic-appearing skin and systemic conditions, and undefined food-associated reactions, i.e., with no elevation of IgE, and to assess TCM effects on these types of conditions.

Using advanced technology to detect pro-inflammatory small molecules, and metabolites to study the underlying mechanisms and monitor the effect of TCM on these conditions.

This research is particularly important for helping bridge the divide between allopathic practice and TCM. At the molecular level, Western science and TCM speak the same language.

Project 5

Clinical observational (anecdotal) study of improvements in general health after treatment with TCM.

This project arose after many parents reported their children were suffering fewer and less-severe colds and other illnesses after beginning TCM treatment. One of the tenets of TCM treatment is that immunomodulation entails up-regulation of Th1-mediated innate immunity, which is associated with resistance to infections, as well as down-regulation of Th2 immunity, tied to allergies. I believe there is a connection with deficient production among allergic people of IgA, which is normally by far the most abundant antibody.[73] People with IgA deficiency are often deficient in making IgG2, making them more allergy and asthma prone.

This inquiry, which is being conducted by a pediatric resident, is interesting because it emerged spontaneously from conversation on social media. As researchers we have to be alert to recognize significant data. A questionnaire is being written to ascertain days lost to school, antibiotic use, asthma exacerbations and use of albuterol, health relative to non-allergic siblings, and other parent testimony.

Other observational studies will be conducted as we continue to accumulate data in practice.

Translational Research

We also have several "bench to bedside" projects, which are supposed to take basic science and seek therapeutic interventions as directly as possible. Such

---

[73] "Common infections observed in symptomatic patients with selective IgA deficiency are recurrent ear infections, sinusitis, bronchitis, and pneumonia," Bellanti, p. 283.

translational projects are necessary to the long-term potential of TCM for many reasons, some of which have already been discussed. That is, to reduce the burden of dosage to even more manageable levels, to put better tools in the hands of allopathic doctors, and in the long run to allow these active ingredients to be synthesized. Growing demand in the face of climate change, land development, and environmental toxicity will strain the available supplies of medicinal herbs.

Project I

Title: To identify bioactive ASHMI™ compounds that act on asthma mechanisms, and develop highly bioavailable versions of them; to identify FAHF-2 compounds that target general allergy mechanisms and then combine these compounds for use in advanced asthma and allergy therapy.

The goal is to develop new super bio-available and long half-life asthma therapies with a daily dose of one pill per day, or even less frequent consumption.

Project II

Title: Development of a natural, pure-compound IgE inhibitor and an inflammation inhibitor.

IgE remains the primary way to keep score for most allergies, despite the recognition and study on non-IgE-mediated allergies. It is especially important for those who have no co-morbid diseases like asthma and eczema, which can be used as markers for "invisible" food allergies. We have already developed a tea called *Xian Cao*, which mothers like to refer to as "IgE tea." We would like to build on this to develop natural, safe, and effective bioactive anti-IgE, anti-inflammatory pure-compound products to treat individuals with multiple food restrictions who are extremely sensitive, and who have had no success in introducing any new foods, or who have been losing tolerance to previously tolerated foods.

Work with translational projects I and II is far enough along, and with sufficient success in clinical practice, that we are already anticipating scaling up production of the pure compounds through creation of a GMP (good manufacturing practices) facility to make quality products in greater quantity.

Project III

Title: A novel mucosal vaccine employing a mucosal adjuvant fused to a major peanut protein, Ara h2, delivered by probiotic spores, BCA vaccine, for preventing peanut allergy anaphylaxis in a murine model.

This is a very different entity from the other research. It is Western science without traditional Chinese medicine. This probiotic is commonly used in Asia for alkaline fermentation of foods. It is designed to create a vaccine that could not only protect individual patients, but possibly reverse intergenerational transmission of a tendency to food allergy. Most of us agree that while allergic tendencies have been around for many centuries, the epidemic we have seen in the past few generations has resulted from relatively recent changes in our environment, diets, and health factors like the gut microbiome. We feel that if these tendencies have been unlocked in a short period, maybe they can be reversed. Henry called this "corrective epigenetics" in his other book. By creating a vaccine, we have a plausible method to do just that.

Clinical observational studies show that children of mothers with peanut allergies or environmental allergies, including allergic rhinitis, have a greater risk of developing peanut allergies than offspring of non-allergic mothers. The balance of Th1, infection-fighting immunity, and Th2, allergic immunity, is skewed toward allergy in these mothers, and they pass this tendency on to their children. Evidence is emerging suggesting that DNA methylation, which tells genes what to do and when to do it, can be modified by dietary and environmental factors and passed on to children. If this can be done in a controlled, safe way, it may be possible to induce maternal tolerogenic epigenetic status and pass this on to the children. However, no such preventive intervention is currently available.

We want to create an oral vaccine for peanut allergies that would have intergenerational benefits. It would employ as an adjuvant non-toxic cholera toxin B (CTB), which has been used safely by pregnant women and infants for 30 years in an oral cholera vaccine. It also induces antigen-specific clinical tolerance in autoimmune disorders when co-administered with antigen by induction of IL-10 and Tregs.

Some people get alarmed when they see the term cholera toxin, which we use to help induce food allergies in mouse studies. However, CTB, a subunit of cholera toxin called cholera toxin-B (CTB) lacks the disease-inducing characteristics of the full toxin. It is the component that first binds to the mucosa and is considered an efficient carrier molecule for generating immune responses to linked antigens, with the added benefit that it possesses immunosuppressing qualities of its own.[74]

CTB's tolerogenic adjuvant activity for vaccinating mothers orally to prevent peanut allergy in offspring has not been previously explored. One problem with any biological medicine that we swallow is to make sure it arrives in the tissue intact, which means surviving the harsh enzymes and acids of digestion. We can use cholera toxin or CTB in mouse studies because we can feed them with a tube. For a human vaccine, we need to find a way of delivering small doses of the allergen and adjuvant to the mucosa in therapeutic quantities.

The vehicle for this is the probiotic bacillus subtilis (BS) spore with the allergen and adjuvant bound to the spore's surface. Spores in nature are very strong, durable, single cell reproductive bodies that germinate new plants such as fungi and algae. They are able to stand up to the hostile digestive environment. This hypothesis is based on previous murine studies showing that maternal allergen immunization of non-atopic mothers prevented their offspring from being sensitized to the allergen. Our own preliminary studies have shown that feeding murine peanut allergy mothers (PA-M) a low dose of peanut antigen together with CTB (PN + CTB), but not peanut alone, during pregnancy and lactation induced tolerance in mothers and prevented allergy in the offspring. An additional hope raised by this research is that because only an extremely low amount of peanut protein is required to elicit a tolerogenic immune response, it may be applicable even to highly sensitive individuals.

---

[74] Antonella D'Ambrosio *et al.*, "Cholera toxin B subunit promotes the induction of regulatory T cells by preventing human dendritic cell maturation," *Journal of Leukocyte Biology* 2008; 84(3): 661–668.

A vaccine that can not only reverse allergy in a mother but reverse the tendency in children would be a powerful weapon in the fight against allergic disease.

Foods that Mimic Health Threats

Parents and doctors speculate constantly about how allergic tendencies have led to an epidemic of food allergies. Mothers especially wonder what they did "wrong." The scientific consensus is that a succession of changes in the way we live, eat, pollute, and medicate result in a cascade of epigenetic changes that make us more reactive to things that are harmless to most people. Adaptive immune responses are largely guided by messages and signaling from the innate immune system. It seems clear that the innate immune system senses something threatening in these allergens that signal the acquired immune mechanism to create antibodies to these things.

What makes the innate immune system mistake these ordinary foods for parasites and other health threats? One very intriguing hypothesis is that the Western diet is mimicking "threat" signals that direct the adaptive immune response away from tolerance and toward arming up to battle perceived dietary threats. Two main avenues for this to happen have been suggested:

One is stimulating release of substances produced by cells that are dying from "non-programmed" causes. They signal the adaptive immune response to join the fight. These substances are called advanced glycation end products (AGE). The Western diet is plentiful in substances that mimic threat signals.

Another avenue is stimulation of enteroendocrine cells that have evolved to "taste" threats — i.e., to perceive them in ways that signals a sensation the way we perceive food when we eat, and if we do not like it to spit it out. One obvious example of this is the TrpV1 receptor in the lungs, which is central to the activation of an inflammatory response to a chemical irritant resulting in an asthma attack. It happens that this is the same receptor that on our tongues reacts to capsaicin, the active ingredient in hot peppers.

Other receptors are T1R, for sweet taste, T2R for bitter, and TRPA1, major oxidant sensor of the body but also a multi-chemoceptor, thermal receptor and ion channel, whose multiple functions make it a powerful agent for mistakenly identifying foods as threats to health.

Highly oxidative and pro-inflammatory diets can stimulate these threat receptors. AGEs are produced in high amounts after eating animal proteins and fats cooked at high temperatures. Fast foods, and particularly bacon, are potent examples. Roasting peanuts, which makes them taste good to most Americans, binds "IgE from patients with peanut allergy at approximately 90-fold higher levels than the raw peanuts" supplied by the same farmers. Excessive sugar in the diet exaggerates AGE signaling to create pro-oxidative stress. Even without research, we can see that much of this data supports what we know about all that is wrong with American diets. We can also see that the cooking methods that produce the effects people like best, such as caramelization during frying or the brown color on a good steak as well as roasting peanuts, produce the worst effects for a whole range of diseases. These are referred to as Maillard reactions. What is new or yet to be researched is how these dietary factors throw the switch toward food allergies specifically.

One obvious approach to studying these mechanisms will be in models of how mice react to a variety of diets, as well as controls whose receptors have been "knocked out" by genetic modification. We know that many of the ingredients of the FAHF-2 mixture work as potent antioxidants and also act as agonists and some mild antagonists of TRPV1 and TRPA1, which would account for its ability to roll back food allergy. A powerful antioxidant called Resveratrol has been shown to block a cholera-induced mouse model of peanut allergy.[75]

We plan to explore several options in murine models. Normal mice with high AGE diet; high AGE with sugar and soda; placebo; and a control for each with the TRPV1 knocked out.

Collaborations

Some of these projects will be done just at Mount Sinai, some in conjunction with my private practice and allopathic allergists, and some in collaboration

---

[75] Y. Okada Y, K. Oh-oka, Y. Nakamura, K. Ishimaru, S. Matsuoka, K. Okumura, H. Ogawa, M. Hisamoto, T. Okuda, A. Nakao, "Dietary resveratrol prevents the development of food allergy in mice," PLoS ONE 7(9): e44338, DOI: 10.1371/journal.pone.0044338.

with distinguished academic researchers in other institutions. For example, testing of the hypothesis that Western diets containing high AGE may contribute to the food allergy epidemic in Western society, and the extent to which FAHF-2 can reverse this process, will be pursued by an international collaborative effort between the Sinai team and an allergist in Australia. I am very happy that our work has attracted so much attention and has begun to excite others who see the potential of reverting to an ancient medical tradition to confront a modern epidemic.

Future of Practice

As Henry wrote earlier, we have begun to take the first steps toward building a practice network, starting with eczema. Mount Sinai, where I work, is also establishing a Center for Integrative Health and Wellness, for which I will serve as Director. This of course follows a wide trend in recent years of mainstream medical institutions to acknowledge and honor patient dissatisfaction with the status quo. This gives us a controlled setting where we can continue to expand the use of our medicines and build expertise in their use through collaboration between allopathic doctors and TCM practitioners without having to educate each in the other disciplines. I did training in both and I believe we do not have to duplicate that career path for everyone. In such a center, practitioners can learn from one another as they go. So much of medicine follows that model anyway. Certainly we have many applicants for clinical and laboratory fellowships.

Future of Supply

In the short run, the challenge will be to deliver medications at doses that recognize human behavior. Too many pills equate with too much non-compliance. We will continue to refine the existing medications so that people will take them at therapeutic levels conveniently and not make excuses or forget.

Beyond this challenge will be the task of meeting demand. My own practice has grown very fast as word has spread through social media. Building a practice network and supplying the new center will add to the strain on supply. Some of the problem is nature itself — plants have growing seasons. Our suppliers have other customers. Therefore, we are working on building our own Good Manufacturing Practices (GMP) facility to make the herbal medicines according to the World Health Organization/Food and Drug Administration standards of purity and potency we have established with our suppliers in China. We must also keep close watch on the market for herbs, which seems to only go up as demand rises. Finally, we must continue to investigate the properties of the active ingredients to plan for the possibility that climate change, pollution, and development will threaten supplies of herbs.

Triple Therapy

An additional study has been planned combining TCM with desensitization using Oral Immunotherapy (OIT) for multiple food allergens and the anti-IgE drug omalizumab. It is hoped that this will bring about rapid tolerance with few adverse events, which are common with OIT alone.

INFORMATION ABOUT DR. LI'S PRACTICE

This is information about Dr. Xiu-Min Li's private practice, adapted from the website liintegrativehealth.com.

1 — Lab Work Required

We will need a copy of your or your child's lab test results before you visit Dr. Li, and we would like to monitor several blood tests every 3–6 months during the traditional Chinese medicine treatment. The lab tests include the following:

Liver function tests: AST, ALT
Kidney function tests: BUN, Creatinine
Total blood counts: white blood cell count, hemoglobin, and platelets
Total IGE to establish a baseline

2 — Conditions Treated

TCM is useful for treating a broad range of conditions that are often grouped under headings like food allergy and asthma, but which may in fact be the result of problems in several organ systems that must be addressed in concert. Bringing about short-term relief and long-term remedy may, under an "integrative" model, be best achieved through a combination of Western medicine in the short run and TCM.

These are conditions that have shown great promise and success in Dr. Li's practice. Others are described in earlier chapters of this book:

1. Frequent GI problems associated with food allergy.
2. Frequent food-induced reactions (once a month or more) and anxiety associated with these reactions.
3. Recalcitrant eczema, associated with daily topical steroid use for more than three months, producing no relief and resulting in depression and diminished quality of life.
4. Asthma, poorly controlled, requiring systemic prednisone at least twice a year, asthma exacerbations twice a month even with inhaled steroids, and daily inhaled steroid use for more than one year.
5. Oral Immunotherapy (OIT) for food allergy patients in both clinical trials and private (non-FDA-approved) treatment who have been forced to drop out because of frequent gastric distress and other adverse reactions.
6. OIT patients in private clinics with GI symptoms who are persisting with treatment but seeking relief.
7. Allergy to multiple foods with peanut and/or nut IgE more than 100KU/L, which is associated with an inability to "outgrow." These are difficult to treat because of the longevity of B memory cells; interpretive TCM approaches may shorten the process of modulating the activities of these cells.

3 — Frequently Asked Questions

1. *What is traditional Chinese medicine (TCM)?*

    TCM has a long history of use in China, Korea, Japan, and other countries, where it is part of mainstream medicine and covered by insurance.

    TCM practice does not focus only on the disease or individual organs. Rather, it addresses establishment and maintenance of the balance of yin-yang (two opposite but complementary forces), the homeostasis of organ systems in the body, and interactions with the environment. The treatment promotes self-healing.

Treatment may be similar if patients have similar symptoms, but usually it is customized for each patient. For example, a "classic" Chinese herbal formulation is a mixture of many herbs, but it can be modified for individual patients depending on the initial combination of symptoms and progress over time.

2. *What is the status of TCM in the United States?*

United States regulators define TCM as a "Whole Medical System" by United States regulators — National Institutes of Health (NIH) and the National Center of Complementary and Alternative Medicines (NCCAM).

TCM is also beginning to play an important role in the US, along with other alternative therapies. Acupuncture needles have been approved by the FDA as medical devices, and are covered by some insurance. Herbal medicines are viewed as dietary supplements and their cost is not covered. However, this is changing. In 1998, the NCCAM/NIH began providing grants to support clinical and basic research on CAM. In 2004, the FDA provided guidance for investigating botanical drug products, including complex formulas containing several herbs, focusing on safety, efficacy, and consistency. Therefore, some dietary supplements may be classified as drugs after completing the clinical trials. In the interim, Flexible Spending Accounts, tax-exempt health care savings accounts, may allow expenditures for alternative medicine.

3. *Why do TCM-based drugs have different names in research and in clinical use?*

The regulatory changes described above created a unique situation. Some investigators began to use Western standard methods to investigate some Chinese herbal medicines with the goal of developing botanical drugs. In parallel with the research, some of these medicines continue to be used in clinical practice as supplements, but they use different names to distinguish them.

Investigational drugs registered with the federal government for research are somewhat different from the herbal formulations used in TCM practices as dietary supplements. The ongoing development process for an investigational drug, or any dietary supplement to gain approval as a drug, is time consuming and very expensive.

4. *What is the goal of TCM treatment for food allergies: desensitization, tolerance, or simply reducing the odds of an anaphylactic response?*

In recent years, an increasing number of publications, including those by Dr. Xiu-Min Li and her colleagues, showed that some constituents of the Chinese herbal medicine formulas suppress IgE production, mast cell and basophil activation, histamine release, and produce beneficial immunomodulatory effects on Th1 and Th2 responses. In animal models of peanut allergy, the herbal treatment produced full protection after seven weeks of treatment, which is the mouse equivalent of 2–4 years of human treatment, and full protection lasted for six months. In the clinic, some multiple food allergic patients passed food challenges one by one after 2–3 years of treatment, and once they passed the challenges they do not relapse with or without regular ingestion.

While it must be noted that these are anecdotal observations and not part of any study, there is ample theoretical reason to believe that the relevant T-helper cells, Th1 and Th2, which govern the immune system, can be re-educated under appropriate conditions and thus effect a "cure."

Th1 is normally the dominant immune response, which protects the individual against bacterial and viral infections and controls the counterpart Th2 response. Th2 promotes IgE production, and activates mast cells/basophils that release histamine and other chemicals which cause allergic symptoms, including anaphylaxis. In food-allergic individuals, Th2 responses become abnormally dominant toward food proteins, leading to over-production of IgE. In general, the severity of reactions in an individual depends upon the amount of food antigen exposure and the extent of mast cell/basophil histamine release. The persistence of food allergy depends on the memory Th2 cells and memory IgE producing B cells/plasma cells.

Therefore, a safe and effective therapy should suppress mast cells/basophil activation and also lower IgE levels, which will reduce reactions. A curative therapy will require re-establishing a Th1 balance that in turn controls the Th2 response and restores a normal immune system, which requires longer treatment.

Does it work? The book *Food Allergies: Traditional Chinese Medicine, Western Science, and the Search for a Cure*, contains several case histories from Dr. Li's clinic, including one about a girl who used to be so sensitive to multiple nuts and had many ER visits, but she is now able to eat them after TCM treatment, and many months after the cessation of treatment.

5. *How will we know the treatment is working?*

This is not an easy question to answer for stand-alone food allergies because it is neither feasible to challenge for food allergies in the short run, nor with any frequency thereafter. Furthermore, it is not practical to test IgE (allergic antibody) levels often; nor are these tests strictly reliable because they measure blood (or serum) IgE levels, not IgE attached to mast cells and basophils, which are the ones responsible for triggering a reaction. However, it is still possible to infer progress if any more visible allergy symptoms are being treated concurrently. For example, relief from eczema is an indicator of diminished allergic activity as is improvement of asthma symptoms.

Other markers to look for: Reduced frequency and severity of reactions. For example, some patients reported frequent reactions, 50 or more, to random exposures, despite careful avoidance. After TCM treatment, the reactions become less severe and less frequent and some patients even have no reactions. Dr. Li says the happiest thing is hearing parents say, "We have nothing to report, everything is quiet." This is a very good sign of improvement.

Food allergies and other immune disorders are quality-of-life conditions (QOL), and any evidence that QOL is improving can be taken as favorable. For example, some children concurrently have asthma and environmental allergies. Improvement of these conditions is also a good sign. Mood-wise, the child becomes happier. Improvement of indigestion, stomachaches, and bowel movement, as well as better overall health, with fewer colds, and other viruses, and sinus infections are all observable outcomes.

It is also important to understand that while first-year IgE levels may not be totally reliable, if blood IgE levels come down to normal or close to the normal levels and are consistent in the following years, you can work with your allergist to do a new round of skin tests and then oral challenges.

6. *What are the herbal bath and herbal cream used for?*

The skin is a very efficient organ for absorbing and distributing the active ingredients throughout the body. Oral dosing has its special role, but when digestion is impaired, as it often is with food-allergic people, the job of processing these compounds is incomplete. Both bath and cream also lower mast cell activity in the skin, which is the largest organ in the body and the primary protection against environmental and infectious toxins. It is uniquely vulnerable to allergen exposure, both by contact and by ingestion. The wide distribution of mast cells throughout this large organ is an important part of the protective effect, but also presents a problem when the immune system has problems as it does with allergies. Finally, the daily oral consumption of a full dose of a variety of herbal medicine can be burdensome, especially for children. It is sometimes difficult to achieve a therapeutic dose. Herbal baths and creams can augment and complement the oral dosing.

7. *What length of time should we expect for treatment?*

This varies according to the individual. It depends on many things, such as age, degree of physical maturity, general health apart from allergies, and many more factors, but a 2–4 year range is a good estimate. As with any medicine, it should not be discontinued at first signs of relief, but Dr. Li has a protocol for tapering off dosage and frequency.

8. *How often will we have to consult with the clinic?*

After the initial consultation, office visits should optimally be scheduled monthly, particularly if acupuncture and/or acupressure are part of the treatment. However, depending on the distances involved — faraway states or countries — the revisits can be arranged typically at 2, 3, 6, or at most 12 months. If long distances are not involved, there should be a consultation approximately every month, either in person or by phone. Email and other non-scheduled consultations are also encouraged, although they should be done judiciously out of respect for Dr. Li's time.

9. *How often do we do blood work and what does it show?*

Total and allergen-specific IgE will be done annually. Complete blood count (CBC) and chemistry tests will be done every six months after reaching full dosing.

Dr. Li's principal concern is that treatment be safe and potentially beneficial. Although TCM therapy itself provided by Dr. Li is very safe, no one can say it is absolutely safe for every patient. Since treatment for immune disorders is a long-term process, Dr. Li likes to see the evidence of safety data. Hence, the requirement for CBC and chemistry lab data at baseline coupled with regular follow-up, because the liver enzyme testing (AST and ALT) can be influenced by behavior and illness. For example, vigorous exercise may increase AST levels. Many medicines such as antibiotics and pain relievers may affect liver enzyme levels. Any abnormalities will elicit more extensive history taking as to activity and illness, and may entail retesting in a few weeks. This does not mean that Dr. Li will not take patients who have abnormal enzyme levels. If the liver enzyme is confirmed to be abnormal, but consistent and there is no underlying condition, she will develop a special TCM protocol to help improve the enzyme levels.

10. *How often are kidney and liver function monitored?*

Kidney and liver function tests are done in the beginning to ascertain whether there are conditions that should be treated on a priority basis, and to avoid the chance, however remote, that the herbal treatments will aggravate them. Because these treatments have a long history of safe use, it is unlikely that they will hurt any organs. Furthermore, the baseline measurements not just of kidney and liver function but other tests will contribute to the body of data accessible to retrospective analysis. After initial panels, they will be done every six months.

11. *Can the clinic order blood work?*

For many reasons, it is preferable for patients to work with their own physicians for things like blood work. On a very practical level, it is easier to get the work reimbursed. For another thing, we welcome collaboration with local physicians to help impart knowledge of TCM that will in the long run contribute to the dissemination of knowledge and achieve the model of integrative medicine. Anyone who needs help persuading a personal physician should contact Dr. Li via the private clinic.

12. *Since so many of us are unaccustomed to this approach to medicine, can you tell us what we should know about what we will face in the months or years ahead?*

Most crucially, because the number of pills is large and because many parents and children have no experience in handling TCM pills, Dr. Li has developed a special protocol for newcomers to further enhance the safety, tolerability and ease.

Dr. Li will ask the family to maintain its day-to-day routine including established food avoidance so that no adverse events take place. Her treatment requires that the body be kept as allergen-free as possible, until all doctors agree that a food challenge is warranted. No self-testing.

If a child has eczema and GI problems, Dr. Li often starts treating these conditions first because they have more day-to-day effect on patient quality of life than food allergies, and because they can be triggered by environmental exposures. Once these conditions are better, Dr. Li will start to treat other conditions.

Dr. Li suggests that you start with one pill first the first morning, and then gradually increase to the full dose. In general the TCM treatment is twice a day. Once the full morning dose is achieved, you can add the evening dose. If more than one regimen is prescribed, you will add them one by one. Most children achieve a full dose at the first month without any sign of problems, but in the event of any problems, Dr. Li will work with you to develop a special protocol. Sometimes other mothers who are very experienced will volunteer to help.

13. *Since many patients, particularly children, are not very adept at taking pills and capsules, can the pills be crushed and added to foods or liquids?*

Yes. These medicines are meant to be ingested as teas, and in the case of some individual ingredients, such as ginger root, are staples of diets throughout the world. They are highly adaptable and can be added to liquids and soft foods. The most important thing is that any mixture be consumed in its entirety. It can be as simple as adding the contents of a capsule or a crushed pill to a couple of ounces of water and a bit of honey for flavor. The most important thing is that these are not chemically delicate medicines, so improvise to suit your child's taste.

14. *Is there a certain amount of time necessary between doses?*

Take as directed. The most important thing is to space the doses by four hours. If the morning dose is missed, it can still be made up by an afternoon and evening dose. However, if you somehow miss two doses by evening, do not take two together before bedtime. Just take one and try to get back on schedule the following day.

15. *What is the digestion tea for?*

As mentioned previously, digestion is often impaired in those with food allergies. In fact, the most allergenic proteins in foods, such as peanuts, are the hardest to digest and are thus most likely to be absorbed intact into the body where they appear to the immune system as threatening invaders. Leaving aside standard diet and medical treatments for the time being, many American digestive systems are in need of repair, and the digestion teas have long track records for achieving this. The tea also helps with constipation, diarrhea, stomachaches, and pains unrelated to allergies.

16. *What side effects should we look for?*

There are no particular side effects, although some patients do have gastric discomfort. This could be the result of adjustment to unfamiliar substances. If these effects persist, they should be described to Dr. Li for possible adjustment of dosing. One of the statistics researchers are most proud of with FAHF-2 is that not a single adverse effect could be attributed to the drug. This is as safe as it gets. There may be other health effects coincident with taking these treatments but they are likely the result of other factors, such as viruses.

17. *Are there long-term side effects?*

No. Dr. Li has seen hundreds of patients, from infants on up, and as long as the protocols are being followed she has seen no complications.

18. *Are there any dietary or activity restrictions during treatment?*

It is only necessary to continue to avoid pertinent allergens for the initial phases of treatment. Activities are permissible, since the whole point of treatment is to achieve a normal existence.

19. *What if my child becomes sick while taking the pills? Do we stop?*

In the case of viruses and bacterial infections that involve vomiting, oral treatment can be suspended, since there is no point in taking medicine that will not stay down. As for baths and creams, it is probably not a good idea to treat the immune system when it is working overtime to fight infection. However, as long as cold symptoms and coughing are not accompanied by fever, there is no reason to stop treatment, and the creams and baths may enhance your child's comfort.

20. *Has anyone ever been allergic to any of the herbs?*

No. Keep in mind that the medicines use herbs in refined form.

21. *What about the inert ingredients?*

Cornstarch is used to bind the active ingredients. Without some form of starch, it would be impossible to manufacture pills. Some people are concerned that they will react to this substance. True corn allergy is very rare. Corn is low in protein to begin with and refining removes almost any conceivable trace of it. For those who have trouble with the starch, special provisions can be made.

22. *What if we miss a dose or two?*

This is a long-term process so missing a few doses here and there, particularly in the case of illness, do not make a significant difference. However, patients should endeavor to stick with their schedules.

23. *Will patients have to take the pills forever?*

The duration of active treatment will not be the same for everyone, and will probably not be "forever." Whether there will be any "boosting" necessary remains to be seen. In mouse trials, diminished protection following cessation of treatment was easily remedied by additional administration of medication. Patients with multiple allergies may see cessation with some faster than with others.

24. *Will taking other medication interfere with taking the herbs?*

Always discuss other medications with all your doctors! Herbal medications do contain active ingredients, and sometimes react with mainstream drugs. Please advise Dr. Li and your physician about all medications, and consult the NIH website:

www.nlm.nih.gov/medlineplus/druginformation.html

With some medicines, there can be synergistic effects. Antihistamines complement the herbal medicines because they block receptors on the IgE attached to mast cells, which inhibits allergic response, while the herbs inhibit production of IgE itself and block histamine release. The combination may be more effective than the herbs alone.

25. *What do the herbs do inside the body?*

They recalibrate an unbalanced immune system toward normal. They do this by moderating the production of allergenic antibodies. Th2 cells, the T-helper cells associated with production of allergic antibodies, or IgE, are "down-regulated" without over-stimulating or damaging other immune function (as is often the case with excessive use of steroidal immune suppressants).

26. *Can the herbs prevent you from getting more food allergies?*

By repairing the digestive system, the herbal treatments make it less likely that allergenic proteins will be absorbed into the system, removing perceived threats, and by down-regulating Th2 IgE output, they reduce reactivity to current allergens. These twin effects make it less likely that new foods will become allergens.

27. *Is it possible to start TCM if we are already participating in another treatment such as OIT or Viaskin™ (the peanut patch)?*

There is no problem in principle because TCM modulates the immune system, instead of desensitizing it to particular allergens, which is the goal of OIT and the patch. It may be that these two processes can complement one another, although that remains to be studied. As a practical matter, however, patients in clinical trials cannot do TCM because it will compromise the study data. Currently, the patch is exclusively being done in trials, and many OIT studies are ongoing. However, patients who are doing OIT in private practice are welcome, provided they are doing it with the cooperation of their treating doctor. For patients who participated in OIT, but stopped because of frequent adverse reactions such as gastrointestinal problems, TCM may be a helpful option.

28. *What are the long-term plans for further research?*

Curative therapy or persistent protection has not been established and the studies of FAHF-2, or a refined version, will carry on. Dr. Li's team continues to make effort and to improve the herbal product for the clinical studies. They developed refined FAHF-2 named B-FAHF-2 (Butanol purified FAHF-2 or B version of FAHF-2). It increases the potency and requires only 1/5 of current FAHF-2 dose to produce complete protection in lab animal model of peanut allergy. For instance, the current version of FAHF-2 requires 36 pills a day for a 12 year old and an adult research subject, but will only need 6 pills of B-FAHF-2 to do the same job. For young child, it will only need 1–2 pills. This refined product will significantly increase the ease of clinical trial. A refined version will be available for clinical practice after an abbreviated safety trial. The refining process will make her clinical TCM supplement products easier to use over a long period of time, reducing the probability of "medication fatigue" and encouraging use for a long enough time with the goal to calibrate the Th1 and Th2 balance and build a healthier immune system.

29. *We have avoided air travel with our child for fear of allergen exposure on airplanes. Is it possible to conduct our consultation via Skype or other online mechanisms?*

The answer is no, for two reasons. First, this has been tried and the technology is just not sufficient. The transmission is halting and not conducive to a fluid conversation. It is not a good use of Dr. Li's time or clinic facilities, especially when there is a waiting room full of patients who have made the trip. Second, the effectiveness of any non-surgical medical therapy is dependent in part on a bond of trust between the patient and doctor. This is especially true in the case of a highly individualized and probably unfamiliar therapy like TCM, which requires daily compliance with a regimen that may include a combination of pills, drinks, baths, and creams. The problem is compounded if acupuncture and/or acupressure are deemed part of the therapy. Skype is just not conducive to establishing the spirit of collaboration among patient, doctor, and parent that comes from face-to-face meetings. While flying has been a source of anxiety for many families, with proper precautions, the risks have been very successfully mitigated by thousands of families. For information on flying with food allergic symptoms, FARE has detailed procedures. http://www.foodallergy.org/managing-food-allergies/traveling

30. *Do the various teas, baths, and creams used in Dr. Li's clinical practice treat specific conditions such as eczema, asthma, and allergies?*

As mentioned, TCM treats the whole patient. The goal is to achieve a healthy, balanced immune system that does not react to allergens introduced via food, contact, or inhalation. Different symptoms in specific organs do not exist in isolation from the rest of the body, and many organs can contribute to a single symptom. Dr. Li chooses not to treat one thing now and another later, unlike Western practitioners who often seek to treat acute problems in isolation from the larger picture. Eczema, or atopic dermatitis, is a prime example. Topical steroids help with inflammation, but without treating the underlying immune system, it will likely return. The same with wheezing and coughing associated with asthma.

There is also the challenge presented by the limitation of any single method of dosing. Medicines introduced by swallowing have the problem of digestion destroying or eliminating a percentage of the active ingredients. Thus, it is necessary to induce additional ones via the skin to achieve a full therapeutic dose. Dr. Li's research shows that multiple molecules contained in these compounds affect multiple other molecules in the body. In this, it is not very different from the discovery of "off label" uses of Western medicines, for example, that a pain reliever like aspirin when used in small doses can stave off clotting and reduce the risk of a heart attack. Thus, FAHF-2 may also prove useful as a treatment for Crohn's disease because of its ability to inhibit secretion of cytokines found in both food allergies and cytokines.

For more information on the science behind Dr. Xiu-Min Li's work, see *Food Allergies: Traditional Chinese Medicine, Western Science, and the Search for a Cure* by Henry Ehrlich (co-author of *Asthma Allergies Children: A Parent's Guide* and editor of asthmaallergieschildren.com).

31. *Many Chinese products, including herbal medicines, have a reputation for contamination with heavy metals and other toxins. How does Dr. Li safeguard her products?*

All extracts and final products must meet official Chinese standards, which are also recognized by the World Health Organization (WHO) Standards of Import and Export of Green Medicinal Plants and Their Preparations, and The State Administration of Traditional Chinese Medicine of the People Republic of China (http://www.satcm.gov.cn/English2010/Policy/2010-10-06/156.html), promulgated by the Ministry of Foreign Trade and Economic Cooperation, the People's Republic of China. Dr. Li uses herbs from areas that are known for purity and are screened for potency of active ingredients. Medicines are tested by the manufacturers, pharmacies at major hospitals, which make all their own drugs right down to saline solutions. All extracts and final products are tested for microbial, pesticide, and heavy-metal residual levels* (Pony Testing International Group in Beijing, an official WHO collaborative lab). Because the US Food and Drug Administration accepts their data, Dr. Li also uses this lab for investigational drugs. Finally, the lab in New York tests for batch quality using certain chemicals markers.

---

*Limited Amount Index: Heavy Metal and Arsenate

Heavy metal content ≤20.0 mg/kg.

Lead(Pb) ≤5.0 mg/kg.

Cadmium(Cd): ≤0.3 mg/kg.

Mercury(Hg) ≤0.2 mg/kg.

Copper (Cu): ≤20.0 mg/kg.

Arsenic(As): ≤2.0 mg/kg.

INDEX

Printed in the United States
By Bookmasters